THE CORTISOL CONNECTION DIET

D0980019

DEDICATION

This book is dedicated to my clients, who over the decade that I've been doing nutritional counseling have taught me as much about metabolic control as I have taught them. It is also dedicated to my wife and best friend, Julie Talbott, who has always been my enthusiastic partner in our own search for control, balance, and happiness in our health and our lives. Thanks.

Ordering

Trade bookstores in the U.S. and Canada please contact:

Publishers Group West
1700 Fourth Street, Berkeley CA 94710
Phone: (800) 788-3123   Fax: (800) 351-5073

Hunter House books are available at bulk discounts for textbook course adoptions; to qualifying community, health-care, and government organizations; and for special promotions and fund-raising. For details please contact:

Special Sales Department
Hunter House Inc., PO Box 2914, Alameda CA 94501-0914
Phone: (510) 865-5282   Fax: (510) 865-4295
E-mail: ordering@hunterhouse.com

Individuals can order our books from most bookstores, by calling (800) 266-5592, or from our website at www.hunterhouse.com

The Cortisol Connection Diet

THE BREAKTHROUGH PROGRAM TO CONTROL STRESS **AND LOSE WEIGHT**

· · · · · · · · · · · ·

Shawn Talbott, Ph.D., FACSM

Hunter House PUBLISHERS

Hunter House Inc., Publishers
PO Box 2914
Alameda CA 94501-0914

Library of Congress Cataloging-in-Publication Data

Talbott, Shawn M.
The Cortisol Connection Diet : the breakthrough program to control stress and lose weight / Shawn Talbott.— 1st ed.
p. cm.   Includes bibliographical references.
ISBN-13: 978-0-89793-450-3 (pbk.)
ISBN-10: 0-89793-450-4 (pbk.)
1. Weight loss. 2. Energy metabolism. 3. Hydrocortisone—Physiological effect. 4. Blood sugar. I. Title.
RM222.2.T28 2003
613.2'5—dc22   2003016844

Project Credits

Cover Design: Brian Dittmar Graphic Design
Developmental and Copy Editor: Kelley Blewster
Proofreader: John David Marion   Indexer: Nancy D. Peterson
Acquisitions Editor: Jeanne Brondino
Editor: Alexandra Mummery
Publishing Assistant: Alexandra Palmer
Publicity Assistant: Gina Kessler
Foreign Rights Coordinator: Elisabeth Wohofsky
Customer Service Manager: Christina Sverdrup
Order Fulfillment: Washul Lakdhon
Administrator: Theresa Nelson
Computer Support: Peter Eichelberger
Publisher: Kiran S. Rana

Printed and Bound by Bang Printing, Brainerd, Minnesota
Manufactured in the United States of America

10 9 8 7 6   First Edition   11 12 13 14 15

Contents

Foreword vii
Acknowledgments ix

Introduction 1

1 Eating for Quality *and* Quantity 6
All Diets Work...for a While 8
Those "Last Twenty Pounds" 9
The Cortisol-Control Approach 11
Quality: What to Eat 12
Quantity: How Much to Eat 15
Two Food Additives to Avoid 17
Timing: When to Eat 21

2 Cortisol Control 27
Why Stress Makes Us Fat 28
Controlling Cortisol Levels 33
Dietary Supplements for Cortisol Control 34
Choosing and Using Supplements Wisely 36

3 Blood-Sugar Control 39
Low-Carb Versus Low-Fat: What to Eat? 39
Why Diets Work 40
The Impact of Insulin 42
The Link Between Cortisol and Blood Sugar 44
The Glycemic Index: Defining Good and
    Bad Carbohydrates 47
Dietary Supplements for Blood-Sugar Control 50

4 Thermogenesis 56
We're Not Getting Any Younger 57

Enhancing Thermogenesis   59
Weight-Loss Supplements to Avoid   63
Dietary Supplements to Enhance Thermogenesis .   65

5 **General Metabolic Support**   74
Thyroid Support   75
Serotonin and Norepinephrine: Natural
    Appetite Control   77

6 **Putting It All Together**   83
Where Does Exercise Fit In?   84
What Type of Exercise Should You Do?   87
Supplements for Optimizing Metabolic Control
    and Weight Loss   89
Sample Menu Plan for Meals and Snacks   91

In Closing   96

A **Putting the Cortisol Connection Diet
to the Test**   97

B **Frequently Asked Questions (FAQ)** 102

Resources 112

Daily Logs 113

Index 128

Foreword

Obesity in America, and indeed in the world, is reaching epidemic proportions. At this writing, more than 65 percent of American adults and nearly one-quarter of our children are overweight or obese. Data from the surgeon general's office have linked more than four hundred thousand premature deaths annually to the direct health effects of obesity (second only to smoking)—and the numbers continue to climb. It is not an understatement that obesity is literally killing America and setting the stage for a national crisis of cardiovascular disease, diabetes, hypertension, and related chronic diseases.

As sports nutritionist for the New York Giants and the School of American Ballet, I see that even professionals can struggle with decisions about what to eat and how to balance their diets. In my private practice, I am active in educating my clients to use diet, exercise, and supplements to help reverse these alarming trends in their own lives. It is evident from the research, as well as from my private practice, that the health effects of obesity can be controlled, that weight can be lost, and that lost weight can be maintained. That recipe for success is expertly presented by Dr. Talbott in *The Cortisol Connection Diet*.

All too often, my clients and health-professional colleagues are confronted with miraculous claims for the latest diet du jour, but rarely do these diets deliver anything but temporary weight loss, inevitable weight regain (and then some), and broken promises. Research from around the world—and practical experience from working with many clients—shows us that lasting weight loss comes from a balanced approach to nutrition, exercise, and responsible supplementation. *The Cortisol Connection Diet* synthesizes many years of this research into a very practical, useful, and easy-to-follow format that will be of tremendous value in helping readers to lose—and keep off—excess weight.

Dr. Talbott bases his Cortisol Connection approach on some of the best research available. He has drawn on evidence from the studies of Dr. Walter Willett at Harvard's School of Public Health and Drs. Rena Wing and James Hill, founders of the National Weight Control Registry. The result is a truly science-based approach to weight loss that uses diet, exercise, and responsible supplementation to control cortisol levels, balance blood sugar, and maximize metabolism.

I think you will find, as I did, that Dr. Talbott's *Cortisol Connection Diet* is a welcome addition to the weight-loss landscape—not only because it is a responsible and science-based approach to weight loss, but also because it is practical, user-friendly, and effective.

— Heidi Skolnik, M.S.
July 2004

Acknowledgments

In setting out to write a "concise" book about harnessing metabolism for weight loss, it rapidly became apparent that conciseness and metabolism have little to do with each other! Just engaging in a discussion of metabolism, especially for people like myself who study it on a day-to-day basis, is like swimming upstream: You can get a good start and put in a noble effort, but it's tough to know when you've gone far enough—or too far. In this regard (knowing where to draw the line in terms of brevity versus detail), I owe a tremendous thank-you to my editors at Hunter House—especially to Kelley Blewster, Jeanne Brondino, and Alexandra Mummery—for helping me to focus my discussion of metabolism on its most relevant aspects.

Introduction

More than two-thirds of American adults—and nearly one-fourth of our kids—are overweight. On any given day, millions of people are using one of the dozens of popular weight-loss programs to help them lose weight. So why do we need another diet?

Low- (and high-) carbohydrate diets, high- (and low-) fat diets, and all manner of high-protein diets promise miraculous results ("Lose 30 pounds in 30 days!" "Lose fat while you sleep!") with little effort ("No exercise!" "No dieting!")—and they're all "guaranteed" to work for you. Almost without exception, these "miracle" diets are more about hype than about offering any real hope of lasting results.

The Cortisol Connection Diet claims only to be a safe, practical, and proven approach that harnesses the three key aspects of metabolism that are at the heart of our epidemic of obesity. Most of all, following the Cortisol Connection Diet will change your metabolic response to food and help you shed those "last twenty pounds" that tend to be the hardest to lose.

As a nutritionist, physiologist, and lifestyle coach for more than a decade, I have used the concepts outlined in *The Cortisol Connection Diet: The Breakthrough Program to Control Stress and Lose Weight* to help thousands of clients optimize their own metabolic profiles—and achieve the lasting weight loss they have been looking for. More often than not, these are people who have tried other diets and have lost weight, but who have had that weight come right back (often with a bit more, as an added "bonus"). Like many of my clients, you may already be following what could be viewed as an excellent diet and exercise plan—but no matter how many calories you cut or how many minutes you exercise, you just can't seem to shed those last few pounds. Sound familiar?

If so, then keep reading. Those last few pounds are the hardest to get rid of because they result from metabolic changes related to blood-sugar and cortisol metabolism. Only by simultaneously optimizing these aspects of metabolism can you realistically hope to achieve your ultimate weight-loss goals—and that is precisely what following the Cortisol Connection Diet can do for you.

When I teach metabolic concepts to my physiology and nutrition students I often use a balloon to illustrate a concept known as *metabolic adaptation*. In this example, I point out that balloons come in a variety of shapes and sizes (just like our bodies), and when we influence one aspect of metabolism (as illustrated by pushing in on the right side of the balloon), we get an equal and opposite reaction in another aspect of metabolism (the balloon swells on its left side). Physicists would refer to this concept as Newton's Third Law of Motion (every action has an equal and opposite reaction), but nutritionists refer to it as metabolic adaptation, and it is one of the overarching reasons why lasting weight loss is so difficult to achieve—unless you know how to use diet and exercise to guide your metabolism in the right direction.

The classic example of how metabolic adaptation applies to weight loss is one in which you cut calories to lose weight, but at the same time your resting metabolic rate (RMR, the number of calories your body burns at rest) also drops—so weight loss continues for a few days or weeks, and then it stops. The weight may even start to creep back onto your hips and belly. This is an example of your body's adapting its metabolism (by burning fewer calories) to its new environment (fewer calories being consumed)—and while the process may have been advantageous for our ancestors' survival when they faced starvation, it doesn't exactly help our weight-loss efforts in the twenty-first century.

The key to lasting weight-loss success is to "outsmart" your body's own process of metabolic adaptation. In other words, you not only need to *think* about the balloon, you need to *be* the balloon! In this context (being the balloon), you need to use what I call the "3-S" approach, which calls for small, simultaneous, and sustained changes in metabolism to help you achieve long-term weight-loss success. The 3-S approach means that you control metabolism just enough to achieve a desired effect (weight loss) but not so much that you cross the line into metabolic adaptation.

By *small*, I mean that we avoid extreme or "big" changes in metabolism, because they set off an almost immediate adaptation that causes our bodies to conserve energy and slow weight loss. Small changes help us to keep "shrinking our balloon"—and most of us want to be smaller balloons.

By *simultaneous*, I mean that we need to influence several different aspects of metabolism at the same time. A significant problem with many popular diets is their inappropriate focus on a single aspect of metabolism—such as appetite control or calorie intake. These are certainly important aspects of any successful weight-loss regimen, but when your diet focuses too much on a single aspect of metabolism, it is very easy for your body to adapt so that it maintains your existing body weight. By contrast, it is much more difficult for your body to fully adapt to small changes made simultaneously in several areas of metabolism.

The Cortisol Connection Diet targets aspects of metabolism that I call *metabolic control points* (MCPs). There are literally hundreds of MCPs that combine and interact in various ways to thwart our weight-loss efforts. They do so by increasing appetite, stimulating fat storage, reducing caloric expenditure, and using many other strategies. Luckily, the scientific evidence is finally offering some clues that we can use to turn the metabolic tables in our favor by addressing the six primary MCPs involved in body-weight regulation: cortisol, blood sugar, thermogenesis, serotonin, thyroid hormones, and norepinephrine. Each of these is addressed in this book.

Finally, by *sustained*, I mean that we need to keep at it. Sometimes this entails changing the plan a bit to stay one step ahead of our own metabolic adaptation. The good news is that the small/simultaneous approach to metabolic control is quite easy to sustain—for life. In fact, most of my clients say they wouldn't go back to their "old" weight-maintenance approaches if I paid them to do so. Why? Simple. Because by following the principles outlined in *The Cortisol Connection Diet*, they look great and they feel great—and who would want to change that?

With the Cortisol Connection Diet, you'll eat all of the foods you love, but you'll learn how to use your food to control the effects of cortisol and glucose (blood sugar) and other MCPs in your body—and ultimately to control how many calories you burn off or store as fat. A special feature of the book is its practical approach to helping you make the Cortisol Connection Diet a part of your everyday life. To this end, I have compiled a series of sample menus and suggestions for dietary supplements in Chapter 6, an extensive list of frequently asked questions (FAQ) about the Cortisol Connection Diet in Appendix B, and easy-to-use daily logs. The logs are provided as a way to get you off to the right start with the Cortisol Connection Diet. You should carry your logs with you during the first few weeks of following the Cortisol Connection approach. The book's small size fits nicely into a purse or a pocket. It will help you to choose foods and meals with a high "balance factor" (more on this later), remind you when to eat and how to supplement your diet, and take the mystery and confusion out of how to approach weight loss. In short, the Cortisol Connection Diet does what other diets fail to do: It emphasizes the practical nature of controlling metabolism in a small, simultaneous, and sustained manner.

The Cortisol Connection Diet is a lasting approach to weight loss because it will show you how to eat for quality and for quantity at every meal. It will show you how to use food, exercise, and dietary supplements to modulate cortisol, blood sugar, energy expenditure, and other aspects of appetite and metabolic control. Following the Cortisol Connection Diet will help you control your appetite, will promote fat loss, and will simply make you feel great—with more energy, better mental focus, and a better body.

If you've been searching for an approach to weight loss that is easy to follow, is based on sound scientific principles, and works for you over the long term, then your search is over. Welcome to the Cortisol Connection Diet.

. . . .
:
.

CHAPTER 1

Eating for Quality
and Quantity

On any given day, millions of Americans are trying to lose weight. In the United States, more adults are overweight than not (65 percent), and almost a quarter of our kids are already overweight (13–24 percent of kids ages six to nineteen) or are rapidly heading in that direction. Forget about "Generation X." Our kids, teens, and adults are on the fast track to becoming "Generation XXL." Estimates from health economists show us that being overweight increases an individual's personal health-care costs by more than six hundred dollars each year, increases the amount he or she will spend on prescription medications by 77 percent, and reduces his or her average life span by about eight years. In many ways, being overweight will either kill you early or put you in the poor house—or both.

Combine all the statistics for the U.S. and they show that more than two hundred million Americans need to lose weight. It is no surprise, then, that we also see hundreds of different weight-loss programs that promise miraculous results to these millions of dieters (and on which we spend, as a nation, more than forty billion dollars each year). Unfortunately, while many of those programs will help people achieve some measure of weight loss, the weight is typically regained in a very short period of time—and almost certainly within a year—after going "off" the diet.

Hundreds of clinical studies show that if you eat in "X" manner, you'll lose weight—but that weight often comes right back, and it comes back more often than it stays off. There are also millions of personal testimonials to support the weight-loss benefits of the various miracle diets, no matter how bizarre they may seem (including all manner of patches, potions, and pills). Without too much effort, it is easy to find diets that promise weight loss by restricting a person's intake of a particular food (such as those "bad" carbohydrates) and others that restrict intake of all foods except those on a certain "approved food list" (which invariably tends to be an arbitrary list with little basis in credible scientific evidence).

It is exceedingly difficult to find anything that a majority of nutrition experts can agree on, but we all generally agree that limiting intake of highly processed grains and sugars can help you keep off the pounds. After that, however, the dietary-advice field becomes a battleground where the debate happens more often in the media than in the laboratory or clinic. No matter what the advocates of the various diets happen to say, the bottom line (for nutrition professionals) comes down to the science. What the science says, quite clearly, is that any of the popular and highly promoted diets can help you lose weight, that they are particularly effective in the early stages of dieting (when you have more than thirty pounds to lose), but that they become less effective for weight loss as get closer to your goal weight. Your choice of diet can also help determine how you might die: Those choosing a high-fat, low-carb diet tend to die of heart disease and stroke, while high-carb, low-fat eaters tend to die of cancer and neurologic diseases.

ALL DIETS WORK... FOR A WHILE

Let's reemphasize one very important fact right here at the start: Virtually *any* diet program will help you lose weight. Whether we're talking about Atkins, Protein Power, Zone, Ornish, Pritikin, South Beach, Paleo, or any of the myriad other choices out there, they will *all* help you lose weight. Why? Because they all restrict total energy intake to about 1,500 calories per day. Do that (restrict calories) on a consistent basis for any length of time (more than a few days), and the vast majority of Americans (or non-Americans eating a "modern American diet") will shed pounds with very little effort.

It's when you get to those last ten or twenty pounds that most diets become less effective—and in some cases actually become counterproductive to your weight-loss efforts. Why? Because most of them target only a single aspect of your metabolism to help you lose weight. And while controlling one aspect of metabolism may be sufficient for the early (easy) stages of weight loss, it becomes woefully inadequate in the later (more difficult) stages—when your weight loss begins to plateau, eventually stops, and often starts to reverse toward weight regain.

For example, the majority of the popular low-carbohydrate diets do a terrific job of helping to modulate blood-sugar levels in people with thirty or more pounds to lose (the "thirty-plus club"—where we find more than 70 million American adults). Through a better modulation of blood-sugar levels, appetite is controlled, fat burning is enhanced, and weight loss follows rapidly for people in the thirty-plus club. (We'll return to the topic of blood-sugar control in Chapter 3.) Unfortunately, just when your low-carb dieting efforts are starting to pay off—and the amount of weight you want to lose falls below twenty pounds (where about 130 million Americans find themselves)—your miracle diet becomes less effective and less miraculous. This is when you hit that dreaded plateau where your previous weight loss of several pounds per week slows to one pound or less per week—and you start the familiar backslide toward weight regain. The same thing can happen on a low-fat diet.

THOSE "LAST TWENTY POUNDS"

This is where the Cortisol Connection Diet comes in. I make no claims that the Cortisol Connection Diet will help you lose *more* weight than Atkins (low carb), or South Beach (low carb), or Ornish (low fat), or any diet in between. But *you'll lose just as much*, and you won't feel hungry or deprived while doing it. However, what the Cortisol Connection Diet will especially do for you (that the others will not do) is help you move beyond the weight-loss plateau where dieters often land when they have twenty pounds to go. It will help rev up your metabolism to get you through the "fifteen to go," "ten to go," "five to go," and "done!" stages of weight loss.

It goes without saying that these later stages are the hardest stages of weight loss—and the ones that cause us the most physical difficulty and mental anguish. Because weight loss gets harder and harder to achieve as we move closer and closer to our goal weight, we need to *simultaneously target multiple metabolic systems* to arrive at our ultimate goal. For the vast majority of us, the metabolic systems that are most tightly associated with those last ten to twenty pounds involve cortisol (the primary stress hormone), blood sugar (which comes into play after meals and at other times throughout the day), thermogenesis (meaning "heat produc-tion" and used as an indicator of your overall metabolic rate and the number of calories your body is burning), serotonin (involved in depression, appetite, and emotional eating), thyroid hormones (key regulators of metabolic rate), and nor-epinephrine (for cellular control of energy levels).

How do I know that the Cortisol Connection Diet will work for you? Because the Cortisol Connection Diet has been studied, and it has been *proven* to work in a group of the toughest cases we could find. These tough cases were people who had tried every popular diet and exercise craze and yet still found themselves with extra weight to lose. They were people who had counted the calories, and the fat grams, and the carb grams—but the weight remained. They were people who had been exercising religiously all along, some of them even partnering with a personal trainer in an effort to "force" those pounds away with extremes of exercise—but again, to no avail: The pounds stayed put. Not until these people joined a study of the Cortisol Connection Diet did they find the solution—and the success—they had been looking for. (If you want to read more about the study, check out Appendix A, "Putting the Cortisol Connection Diet to the Test.")

Stephanie

To be honest, before trying Dr. Talbott's program, I had almost given up on my goal to lose twenty-five pounds. I was already running for an hour on most days and doing other exercises when I could, but I just couldn't seem to lose the weight. It's like Dr. Talbott says: "Exercise alone won't work." It wasn't until I put together all the pieces of the complete program that the pounds and belt notches began to drop. If I had never found Dr. Talbott's program, I wouldn't have the knowledge I needed to be successful, and I never would have reached my weight-loss goal.

By using Dr. Talbott's helping-hand and balance-factor approaches to eating I was never hungry, I had no cravings, and I never felt like I was on a "diet" of any kind. By following this program, I have made a

complete 180-degree turn with my eating habits—
and these changes have benefited my family as well
as me. Now we all have healthier eating habits and
better energy levels. The best part of the plan, however, is the stress relief that comes from following the
guidelines. By remembering Dr. Talbott's words about
stress eating and cortisol, I was able to stop stressing
out about food. The real blessing is that this stress
relief also worked its way into my daily life. I am now
happy with myself and with the people around me,
and I was able to stop taking antidepression medication without any problems. My husband can't stop
commenting on the "new me."

I am so thankful for the knowledge and information I have gained from following Dr. Talbott's program. It has moved my life, and the lives of my family, in a positive and healthy direction. I know that if I
hadn't found Dr. Talbott's program, I would not have
lost the extra weight I was carrying around, because I
had already tried on my own many times. The Cortisol
Connection Diet is priceless! Thank you, Dr. Talbott!

THE CORTISOL-CONTROL
APPROACH

The Cortisol Connection Diet is not about following a strict
meal-planning regimen, nor is it about restricting any foods
or categories of foods. In fact, it's not much of a "diet" at all.
Most of the people who have tried it can confirm that they
often eat *more* food while following it—and they still lose
weight. The Cortisol Connection Diet teaches you how to
balance your intake of carbohydrates, protein, fat, and fiber in
a way that considers both the quantity of food (as all weight-
loss diets must do) and, even more importantly, the quality of
those foods. The term *balance factor* (also known as the *balance index*) refers to the quality/quantity of foods and meals.

Specifically, *quality* refers to what you eat, and *quantity* refers to how much you eat. Don't worry about trying to stick to eating only certain items from a long list of "approved" foods (because all foods are fair game) or avoiding other foods on some "banned" list (because no foods are prohibited).

Figuring out the balance factor for a particular food is easy—and generally follows a simple three-step "quality analysis" that you can do when choosing foods at the grocery, selecting a sandwich at the deli, or ordering a meal from a restaurant menu.

QUALITY: WHAT TO EAT

Step 1—Consider Carbohydrates

General rule: Foods that are more "whole" (in their natural, unprocessed state) have a higher balance factor.

Carbohydrates, in and of themselves, are not "bad," but the form of carbohydrate that you choose will determine your body's metabolic response and your likelihood of storing that food as fat. Here are some examples of this principle in action:

- A whole apple is less processed than applesauce, which is less processed than apple juice—so the apple has the highest balance factor, applesauce is moderate, and apple juice is low.

- All whole fruits and vegetables have a high balance factor, and thus can be used to "balance" a food that has a lower balance factor (such as a juicy Italian sausage sandwich at the company picnic—see below).

- Whole-grain forms of high-carbohydrate foods have a higher balance factor than forms that use highly refined grains. When choosing breads, pastas, and crackers, always look at the label for "whole-grain flour" or "whole-wheat flour" and choose the products that contain them instead of products that simply state "wheat flour," which indicates a more highly refined grain rather than a whole grain.

◆ When you don't have a label to consult (such as when eating out), choose grain products that are thicker, chewier, and heartier—such as "peasant breads," with added seeds, nuts, and fruits—rather than "fluffier" and "softer" breads, which indicate highly refined grains.

◆ Choosing whole, unrefined fruits, vegetables, and grains over processed versions of these foods will naturally boost your fiber intake, another important part of the balance-factor approach to eating (see Step 4, below).

Step 2—Provide Protein

General rule: Any form of lean protein can be used to "rebalance" a refined carbohydrate.

◆ Protein and carbs are the "yin and yang" of nutrition: They have to be consumed together for proper dietary balance (which falls apart when either one is excluded or inappropriately restricted).

◆ Leaner sources of protein are always a better choice than fattier cuts (choose 97 percent lean ground beef instead of 85 percent lean).

◆ A bagel for breakfast is not necessarily a "bad" carbohydrate, but it has a low balance factor (especially if it's made from refined, white flour instead of whole-wheat flour) until you add some protein—perhaps in the form of smoked salmon or a scrambled egg. The combination of a high-balance-factor food (virtually any protein) with a low-balance-factor food (a refined-grain bagel) balances the meal into one with a "moderate" balance-factor profile—and it is these "moderate" balance-factor meals that will make up the majority of what you will eat while on the Cortisol Connection Diet.

◆ Some foods might masquerade as protein—such as bacon, sausage, hot dogs, kielbasa, cheese, nuts, and peanut butter—but their very high fat content means that we treat them as "added fat" and consider how they affect our balance factor in Step 3.

Step 3—Finish with Fat

General rule: A small amount of added fat at each meal is a "metabolic regulator."

◆ A bit of added fat—in the form of a pat of butter, a dash of olive oil, a square of cheese, or a handful of nuts—helps to slow the postmeal rise in blood sugar, which in turn helps you control appetite and enhances fat burning throughout the day.

◆ Your choice of pasta as a side dish (but not as a main meal—see quantity discussion in the next section) is an "okay" choice, with a low to moderate balance factor. You can raise its balance factor by choosing whole-grain pasta (instead of the typical highly refined forms) and/or by topping it with a delicious olive oil, garlic, and basil sauce. Even better, mix some fresh vegetables into the sauce to further boost the balance factor of the entire meal.

◆ Your child's lunch of white bread with grape jelly is a low-balance-factor disaster (you might as well inject sugar straight into her veins and fat into her adipose tissue), but you can boost the balance factor of her sandwich by adding a bit of peanut butter, insisting that she wash it down with a glass of 1 or 2 percent milk, and switching to whole-wheat bread (a tough switch with many kids, but well worth the try).

Step 4—Fill Up with Fiber

General rule: Choosing "whole" forms of vegetables, fruits, and grain (as recommended in Step 1) will automatically satisfy your fiber needs.

Like fat, fiber helps to slow the absorption of sugar from the digestive tract into the bloodstream. In this way, fiber can also be considered a "metabolic regulator" that helps balance blood-sugar levels at each meal or snack. The fiber content of whole foods also provides a great deal of "satiety"—that is, foods high in fiber make us feel fuller for longer, so we are less likely to feel hungry. Part of the reason why high-balance-factor carbohydrates are considered beneficial is due to their higher fiber content and the resulting blood-sugar control.

QUANTITY: HOW MUCH TO EAT

At the same time that you are evaluating the quality aspects of your food choices, you should also be considering the second part of the balance factor: quantity (otherwise known as "portion control"). When we talk about quantity, we know without a doubt that size matters! Luckily, Mother Nature was looking out for your waistline when she equipped you with a handy pair of built-in portion-control devices. You probably know them as your hands. This fortunate fact means that we have no excuse to overeat, because we can use our hands to guide us in the quantity part of the Cortisol Connection Diet. It works like this:

Carbohydrates

General rule: Whenever possible, select higher quality carbohydrate sources—but only eat a certain quantity of them (see below).

Fruits and vegetables (except potatoes)— Choose a quantity of fruits and vegetables that roughly matches the size of your open hand. Select brightly colored fruits and vegetables for the highest levels of disease-fighting carotenoids (orange, red, yellow) and flavonoids (green, blue, and purple).

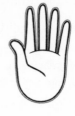

Starches, i.e., bread, cereal, pasta, and other concentrated carb sources (including potatoes and French fries)—Choose a quantity that is no larger than your tightly closed fist (a small side dish of pasta, potato salad, a dinner roll, etc.).

Protein

General rule: Whenever possible, avoid consuming carbohydrates (of any quality level) without added protein and fat.

Lean proteins, such as those found in eggs, low-fat yogurt, skim or low-fat milk, 97 percent lean ground beef, steak (with visible fat trimmed), fish (any), chicken (breast is best), pork chops, etc.—Choose an amount that approximately matches the size of the palm of your hand. (Note that I said palm. I am not referring to your entire open hand.) Keep in mind that this portion is likely to be only about half of the size of the standard portion served in many American restaurants—so be prepared to eat half and bring the other half home for leftovers.

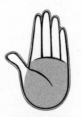

Fat

General rule: Whenever possible, avoid consuming carbo-hydrates (of any quality level) without added protein and fat.

Any source of fat will do (except most mar-garines—see below). That means butter, olive oil, flaxseed oil, canola oil, cheese, and nuts are fine. Make an okay sign with your thumb and index finger, and choose an amount of fat about the size of the circle made between your index finger and thumb.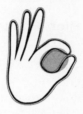

The above "helping-hand" approach to eating considers both the quality and the quantity of every meal and snack—and the best part is that it requires zero counting of calories, fat grams, or carb grams. Why? Because the calorie control is already built in, based on the size of your hands (Mother Nature's automatic portion control device). That means a person with average-sized hands (and likely an average-sized body and metabolism) will consume about 500 calories from each meal built using the balance-factor hand approach. Smaller individuals (with smaller hands and metabolic rates) will have smaller meals of approximately 400 calories each, while larger people (with larger hands and metabolic rates) will have larger meals that come closer to 600 calories each. Eat this way at breakfast, lunch, and dinner and you'll con-sume about 1,200 to 1,800 calories—or precisely the same range of calories associated with the very best long-term weight-loss success.

TWO FOOD ADDITIVES TO AVOID

I mentioned at the beginning of the chapter that the Cortisol Connection Diet has no "banned foods" list. However, there are two food additives that have such a low balance factor as to actually be negative and therefore impossible to balance with even the highest-balance-factor foods. These ingredients are high-fructose corn syrup and hydrogenated or partially hydrogenated vegetable oils.

High-Fructose Corn Syrup

High-fructose corn syrup (HFCS) is a sweetener made from corn. HFCS is higher in fructose than regular corn syrup or table sugar, which is technically known as *sucrose*. (By the way, sucrose is hardly better than HFCS because it is 50 percent fructose and 50 percent glucose.) The food industry likes to use HFCS to sweeten processed foods because it is both cheaper and sweeter than regular sugar, so they can use smaller amounts of it and save money. The food industry is not alone in its love of fructose. We, as consumers, also love fructose, as evidenced by the 26 percent increase in our per capita consumption of it, from 64 grams per day in 1970 to 81 grams per day in 1997. Some subsets of the population, such as teenagers, consume more than 100 grams a day per capita (largely due to their high intake of processed foods and soft drinks).

If nothing else had changed in our diet or lifestyle, this 17-gram increase in fructose consumption would result in a relatively minor increase in energy consumption of 68 calories per day—certainly not enough to account for the epidemic increase in the number of Americans who are overweight. However, because fructose is metabolized quite differently from other sugars, overconsumption of it can result in some very dramatic alterations in energy metabolism, including disrupted cortisol metabolism in fat cells, which encourages them to store more fat in abdominal fat depots (that is, in the belly).

Several animal studies and some recent human studies have suggested that HFCS leads to many of the same metabolic changes that in turn lead to obesity, such as insulin resistance, increased appetite, lower leptin levels (which further increases appetite), and others.

Leptin—from the Greek *leptos*, meaning "thin"—is a hormone with important roles in regulating appetite, body weight, metabolism, and reproductive function. Insulin is the hormone responsible for delivering energy, in the form of glucose, or blood sugar, to the body's cells. A person who is insulin resistant has cells that respond sluggishly to the action of insulin; thus, that person will tend to have trouble regulating blood-sugar levels, body weight, and overall metabolism.

Because fructose does not increase levels of insulin and blood sugar as quickly as sucrose and glucose do, it has been recommended in the past as a sweetener for diabetics needing better blood-sugar control. Unfortunately, while we certainly don't want blood sugar or insulin levels to rise excessively, we do want them to rise moderately following a meal, because this is a potent signal to the brain to cut appetite. Without a rise in blood sugar, leptin, and insulin following a meal, the brain never receives this important signal to stop eating, and we continue to be hungry. In a landmark study published in 2002 in the *American Journal of Clinical Nutrition*, researchers from the University of California at Davis showed that a high level of fructose in the diet was a "significant factor determining the likelihood of weight gain" because of the effect of fructose in disrupting this important appetite-signaling system.

The bottom line with fructose, especially as HFCS in processed foods, is that when we eat it, we get the calories, and we get the signal to store those calories as fat, but we don't get the satiety signal that tells us to stop eating. In theory, you could gulp down a six-pack of cola sweetened with HFCS and not even "register" that you had consumed those calories (though your waistline would certainly have no problem storing them as fat).

Hydrogenated Oils

Hydrogenated oils are liquid vegetable oils that have been chemically modified (by pumping extra hydrogen atoms into their chemical structure) to take on a solid or semisolid form. Think Crisco or other vegetable shortenings. These hydrogenated oils, also called *partially hydrogenated oils*, *trans-fats*, or *trans-fatty acids* (which refers to the change in their chemical structure), are easier to handle than liquid oils during food processing, and are preferred in many processed foods because they can add crispiness to crackers and longer shelf life to cookies. The downside for our health is that trans-fats can also increase LDL cholesterol (the "bad" kind), reduce HDL cholesterol (the "good" kind), and increase systemic levels of inflammation in the body (setting the stage for cardiovascular disease).

When it comes to your weight, hydrogenated oils contribute the same 9 calories per gram as nonhydrogenated forms of fat, but it's the way they are metabolized in the body that is important. Trans-fats are known to interfere with the metabolism of cortisol (increasing cortisol levels), blood sugar (increasing blood glucose and inhibiting insulin function), and the inflammatory cascade (nudging it toward a proinflammatory state, which further interferes with cortisol metabolism). The overall effect of a diet high in trans-fats is to deliver a potent signal to adipose tissue cells (i.e., fat cells) to store as much fat as possible and release as little as possible, even when calorie intake is cut way down.

The bad news is that both trans-fats and HFCS are found in high amounts in many processed foods—but the good news is that they are highest in low-balance-factor "junk" foods that you'll already be limiting as part of the quality portion of your Cortisol Connection Diet approach to eating. As a general rule of thumb, any food that lists either of these additives as one of the first three ingredients on its label should automatically be considered a *negative*-balance-factor food and should not be part of your diet.

There are many excellent studies and books covering the scientific evidence concerning the wide-ranging health effects of these additives on cardiovascular health, hormone regulation, brain biochemistry, and, of course, body-weight regulation. For readers interested in a detailed overview, I refer you to the extensive discussions of these additives and their health effects found in the books by Harvard University's Dr. Walter Willett and the University of Arizona's Dr. Andrew Weil (listed in the Resources).

TIMING: WHEN TO EAT

The last aspect of the Cortisol Connection Diet to discuss is timing, or when to eat. The Cortisol Connection approach represents a subtle but important departure from many popular diets. The Cortisol Connection Diet, like many existing programs, encourages you to eat several small meals and snacks throughout the day. This approach to eating can do wonders for helping to modulate your blood-sugar and cortisol responses to food, thereby helping to control appetite, boost energy levels, and encourage fat burning throughout the day.

The Cortisol Connection Diet optimizes this approach by spacing out three meals and three snacks throughout the day in the following pattern:

7 A.M.   Snack (before leaving for work)

9 A.M.   Breakfast (at work)

Noon   Snack (plus exercise if you can fit it in)

2 P.M.   Lunch

5 P.M.   Snack (before leaving work or on the way home)

7 P.M.   Dinner (with a cocktail or a small dessert as your optional fourth "snack" of the day)

A snack consists of one appropriately sized serving from the fruit/veggie group, plus one appropriately sized serving of fat (such as an apple and a piece of cheese). A meal consists of one appropriately sized serving from each of the starch, protein, and fat groups, plus one or two appropriately sized servings from the fruit/veggie group.

Note: From a weight-loss perspective, a snack can consist of one serving from any of the groups, but from an overall health perspective, it is better if the snack consists of one serving from the fruit/veggie group plus one serving of fat. This combination delivers more fiber and important phytonutrients that are less likely to be found in a protein or starch serving (though whole-grain starches would not be a bad second choice, because they also contain phytonutrients such as lignans).

You'll notice that each snack "lasts" for two hours and each meal "lasts" for three hours. The snacks and meals are spaced out in this manner because I have found it to work the best for the majority of the busy professionals who come to me for nutrition consultation and diet design. Not many of us are able to sit down to a relaxing breakfast before heading out the door for work; it's usually something scarfed from the drive-through on the way to rush-hour traffic. Likewise, most of us aren't able to be home from work with enough time to watch the evening news, prepare dinner, and enjoy a meal anytime before seven at night. This schedule also worked very well for the participants in our twelve-week study of the Cortisol Connection Diet. It led many of them to remark that they felt like they were "always" eating and "never" hungry and yet still losing fat and inches. In this scenario, your snacks act as "bridges" between meals and as significant controllers of cortisol, blood sugar, and overall metabolic rate. Do not neglect them!

Chapter 6 brings everything together with examples of what high-balance-factor meals and snacks might look like. Use it to guide you in crafting your own balance-factor approach to effective, long-lasting, and tasty weight loss.

The back of the book includes blank daily logs to help get you off to the right start with the Cortisol Connection Diet. You should carry your log with you during the first few weeks of following the Cortisol Connection Diet approach (the book's small size fits nicely into a purse or a pocket). It will help you to choose foods and meals with a high balance factor, remind you when to eat and how to supplement your diet, and take the mystery and confusion out of how to approach weight loss.

That's it. At this point, you can see how the balance-factor approach to eating can be easy to follow, practical to use in your everyday life, and effective as a way to control the key aspects of metabolism that are keeping many of us from losing those last ten to twenty pounds. The next four chapters focus on the specific metabolic factors that cause most of us to gain weight and struggle with weight loss. Those factors are cortisol, blood sugar, thermogenesis, serotonin, thyroid hormones, and norepin-ephrine—and all six are wonderfully controllable by eating in the balance-factor way and prudently adding specific dietary supplements to enhance metabolic control.

Chapter Highlights

◆ The Cortisol Connection Diet can help you lose just as much weight as other popular diets, without unnecessary restrictions, counting calories, or counting grams of fat or carbs.

◆ The Cortisol Connection Diet is the only program that simultaneously addresses the six aspects of metabolism that are most tightly associated with the loss of those "last ten to twenty pounds." These are

1. cortisol (the primary stress hormone),

2. blood sugar (which comes into play after meals and at other times throughout the day),

3. thermogenesis (meaning "heat production" and used as an indicator of your overall metabolic rate and the number of calories your body is burning),

4. serotonin (involved in depression, appetite, and emotional eating),

5. thyroid hormones (key regulators of metabolic rate), and

6. norepinephrine (for cellular control of energy levels).

◆ Only by simultaneously optimizing these multiple aspects of metabolism can you realistically hope to achieve your ultimate weight-loss goals.

◆ The balance-factor approach to eating encourages weight loss by balancing your intake of high-quality carbohydrates, protein, fat, and fiber. When it is combined with the helping-hand approach to quantity (portion) control, you eat approximately 500 calories at each meal—leaving you with a low-stress and high-enjoyment form of meal balancing.

◆ Other benefits of the Cortisol Connection Diet besides weight loss include:

— less tension

— better mental focus

— more restful sleep

— fewer/reduced cravings

— enhanced stamina

— general feelings of well-being

Jenni

The last three months have changed my life and my family members' lives. I will never go back to the person I was after being on Dr. Talbott's Cortisol Connection Diet program. When I received the phone call from my girlfriend telling me about the three-month program, I was thrilled. I was a very frustrated person, seeking answers and not getting them anywhere!

I am a thirty-five-year-old mother of five and thirty-five pounds overweight. I have always been active and started running seven years ago. At that time I had no problem with my weight. About five years ago I found myself struggling to keep my weight where it needed to be. I increased my daily running to five miles a day, five days a week, and even that didn't work—I still kept gaining weight. I started eating only three times a day, with no snacks and nothing after 6:00 P.M., and that only made me hungry, tired, and frustrated because I gained even more weight. Then I started looking up all the popular diets, but they all seemed so strict and unforgiving, and I knew that I could never last on any of them. I was seriously in trouble and knew I needed help but didn't know where to go or what to try next. Dr. Talbott's program answered all my questions. It not only helped me lose the weight, but it also actually changed my life forever because of how I (and my entire family) feel. We're happy, excited, energetic, and full of life. I will tell everybody that I know about how Dr. Talbott's program changed my life and gave me back the energy that I hadn't felt in years. Thank you, thank you, thank you for sharing this with me.

. . . .
      .
      .

CHAPTER 2

Cortisol Control

I f you could change one aspect of your life that would give
you the greatest chance of becoming thin and living to a
hundred, what do you think it should be? Fat intake? No.
Exercise level? No. Vitamin supplements? No.

The correct answer is to reduce your stress level. If we
look at the predominant lifestyle factors among people who
have cracked the century mark, we see that they are at their
ideal body weight and that they share what psychiatrists call a
"lack of neuroticism." The ability to handle stress well and to
avoid obsessing about their troubles helps these centenarians
stay feeling great because these tendencies help them balance their cortisol levels, maintain their immune-system
function, and keep their metabolic rate humming.

There is no doubt that we live in stressful times, whether
our stress comes from traffic jams, office deadlines, kids,
spouses, in-laws, bills, or any of the other stressors that come
with a modern lifestyle. These are all forms of chronic stressors that many of us are faced with on a daily basis. Another
one, believe it or not, is the mental stress that accompanies
dieting and worrying about your weight.

As a culture, we're finally catching on to the notion that
managing stress and cortisol levels can extend our lives, help
us lose weight, and generally make us feel better in many
ways. Since 1998, the number of Americans practicing yoga
has jumped by more than 300 percent. That means that over

fifteen million of us are humming, stretching, and breathing our way to healthier cortisol levels. According to a study by business consultant PricewaterhouseCoopers, stress relief is turning into a big business—with the number of spa visits up 71 percent from 1999 to 2001 (at an average of seventy dollars per visit).

WHY STRESS MAKES US FAT

Clinical studies from Yale University, the University of Miami, the University of California at San Francisco (UCSF), the University of Connecticut, the University of Chicago, and many others around the world have shown that lowering stress levels and returning cortisol levels to normal can reduce body-fat levels, control blood pressure, improve insulin sensitivity, balance blood-sugar levels, and control appetite. The best news is that numerous studies have shown that yoga, massage, exercise, eating right, and using certain dietary supplements can all deliver an antistress and cortisol-controlling benefit in a variety of stressful circumstances—so you have lots of choices for getting your stress and cortisol levels under control.

Stress leads to weight gain primarily because of cortisol, the body's main stress hormone. When we're under chronic stress, the amount of cortisol circulating in our body stays elevated. Cortisol acts as a potent signal to the brain to increase appetite and cravings for certain foods, especially carbohydrates and fats (because of their high calorie levels). Cortisol also acts as a signal to our fat cells to hold on to as much fat as they can and to release as little fat as possible, even in the face of our attempts to reduce calorie intake for weight loss. If that weren't already bad enough for our weight-loss efforts, cortisol also slows the body's metabolic rate by blocking the effects of many of our most important metabolic hormones,

including insulin (so blood-sugar levels suffer and carb cravings follow); serotonin (so we feel fatigued and depressed);
growth hormone (so we lose muscle and gain fat); and the
sex hormones testosterone and estrogen (so our sex drive
falls and we rarely feel "in the mood" when we're stressed out
and awash in cortisol).

All these metabolic factors combine when we're under
stress to create a situation in which we eat more food, burn
fewer calories, and store more fat. This isn't good! In terms
of weight gain, the link between cortisol and deranged
metabolism is seen in many ways. Some of these are listed in
the box on page 30.

All in all, the discouraging truth is that stress makes us
fat. Even worse news, however, may be the findings from
researchers who have determined that the "stress" of dieting
can also keep us fat by making it harder for us to lose weight
and easier for us to regain any weight that we *do* lose. Why is
this especially bad news? Because at any given moment, as
much as 50–60 percent of the population is actively dieting—
and many millions more are at least concerned about what
they eat. This makes dieting one of the most common stress
triggers in our modern society, for both men and women.

During periods of chronic stress, such as when dieting,
rising cortisol levels send a potent signal to fat cells, telling
them to store as much fat as possible. Cortisol also signals fat
cells to hold on to their fat stores; therefore, stress can actually reduce the ability of the body to release fat to burn for
energy. Does this mean that people with higher levels of stress
are less able to lose weight? Yes—for a variety of reasons.

In one study, volunteers took part in a fifteen-week
weight-loss program. They were put on a diet of 700 calories
per day. As expected, they experienced a significant increase
in overall hunger, desire to eat, and total food consumption
(when they were finally allowed to eat as much as they

Metabolic Effects of Elevated Cortisol (Related to Weight Gain)

Loss of Muscle Mass

- Breakdown of muscles, tendons, and ligaments (to provide amino acids for conversion into glucose)
- Decreased synthesis of protein (to conserve amino acids for conversion into glucose)
- Reduced levels of DHEA, growth hormone, IGF-1, and thyroid-stimulating hormone (TSH)
- Drop in basal metabolic rate (i.e., a reduced number of calories is burned throughout the day/night)

Increase in Blood-Sugar Levels

- Reduced transport of glucose into cells
- Decreased insulin sensitivity
- Increase in appetite and carbohydrate cravings

Increase in Body Fat

- Increase in the overall amount of body fat (due to increased appetite, overeating, and reduced metabolic rate)
- Redistribution and accumulation of body fat in the abdominal region

Bottom line:
Cortisol blocks your weight-loss efforts.

wanted). It turned out that the most consistent predictor of these increases in desire and consumption was the change (increase) in cortisol levels due to the stress of dieting. The researchers hypothesized that the low-calorie diet induced a form of stress that raised the subjects' cortisol levels and caused them to eat more. Another study exposed a group of women to both a "stress session" and a "nonstress" (control) session on different days. The women who reacted to the stress by secreting higher levels of cortisol were the very same women who consumed more calories on the stress day compared to the low-stress day. Also of note was the fact that the women producing the most cortisol were not only hungrier, but they also showed an increase in negative moods in response to the stressors (which were significantly related to food consumption). These results suggest that stress-induced elevations in cortisol levels can strongly influence eating behavior, emotional outlook, and body weight.

In study after study, we see that elevated cortisol levels lead to increases in body fat—whether the stress comes from a lack of sleep (as in studies from the University of Chicago), mental pressure (as in studies from Yale, Stanford, and the University of California at San Francisco), or socioeconomic status (as in studies from Goteberg University in Sweden). One of the most compelling findings about the relationship between stress, cortisol, and weight gain, however, comes from two studies of young women by researchers at Yale University and the University of British Columbia. In these studies, the women with high levels of "cognitive dietary restraint" (meaning that they put a lot of mental energy into restricting themselves from eating certain foods) had significantly higher cortisol levels, bigger appetites, increased consumption of sweets, more negative moods, and higher body-fat levels—despite also getting more exercise (which would tend to reverse these findings). In animal studies from the

University of Medicine and Dentistry of New Jersey (UMDNJ), stressed-out rats had cortisol levels that were 48 percent higher than nonstressed rats, and they ate 27 percent more and became 26 percent fatter.

Researchers at the University of Colorado have shown that athletes who exercise too much (overtrained cross-country skiers in the case of this study) experience the very same adverse effects of elevated cortisol levels, such as mood disturbances, immune-system suppression, and increased levels of body fat. Of particular interest in this study was the finding that the athletes who were working out the most—those putting in the highest mileage and the longest training times—were also the ones with the highest cortisol levels, the highest body-fat levels, and the poorest scores on measures of emotional outlook (more depression). Basically, they were exercising their brains out to get into better shape, but their elevated cortisol levels were hampering, and indeed outright preventing, their progress.

Sandy

I might be the "perfect" candidate for Dr. Talbott's Cortisol Connection Diet because I am the stereotypical stress eater. I started Dr. Talbott's program during a very stressful time for me—and I expected to gain weight as usual because of the stress. My husband is out of town for work at least three or four days each week, so I basically have no break between work, kids, and everyday stresses. But Dr. Talbott's program was so simple to follow that it actually made things easier to handle (instead of harder to follow, as is the case with many other diets I have tried). I have always been a "tough case" when it comes to weight loss— as soon as I gain it, the weight just stays there on my hips and waist. But with Dr. Talbott's program the weight and inches just started to come off without any real attention from me. The program has taught me so much about nutrition and metabolism and how important it is to do several small things at one time to control weight. The most noticeable effect for me was to eat small meals and snacks during the day to help control blood-sugar levels—it worked so well that I never had cravings.

I am thankful that I was finally able to find the waist that my "middle-age-spread" had erased. It's great to wear jeans again and not have bulges over the top and out the front. No baggy tops for me anymore. I will forever be a believer in Dr. Talbott's program and I will tell all my friends about it!

CONTROLLING CORTISOL LEVELS

So where does this leave us? In terms of weight loss, we know quite clearly that stress, excessive dieting, and cortisol are all detrimental to our overall goals of shedding extra body fat. We also know from decades of research that appropriate levels of exercise and proper diet can be helpful in controlling stress, cortisol, body weight, and a whole host of related health parameters. For a complete cortisol-control regimen, I refer you to my previous book on the topic, *The Cortisol Connection: Why Stress Makes You Fat and Ruins Your Health— and What You Can Do about It* (Hunter House, 2002), which discusses cortisol metabolism in great detail and presents an overall cortisol-controlling regimen called the SENSE program. SENSE incorporates practices of Stress management, Exercise, Nutrition, Supplementation, and Evaluation to help you modulate cortisol levels.

For right now, however, you can keep reading this book, because the Cortisol Connection Diet incorporates the nutrition aspect of the cortisol-control program by balancing the quality and quantity of the foods you'll consume at each meal. The exercise portion is covered in Chapter 6, and information on supplementation follows in the next section.

DIETARY SUPPLEMENTS FOR CORTISOL CONTROL

When it comes to dietary supplementation for cortisol control, the first line of defense comes in the form of a comprehensive multivitamin/multimineral supplement. The most effective choices are products that offer a balanced blend of the key vitamins and minerals that the body needs in order to mount an appropriate stress response. In particular, vitamin C, calcium, magnesium, and the full B-complex group are of the highest importance from the standpoint of their direct involvement in the body's stress response, but all of the essential and semiessential vitamins and trace minerals are needed as well. A comprehensive multivitamin/multimineral supplement, when used as part of a regimen of balanced diet and regular exercise, represents the antistress foundation on which you can add the targeted cortisol-control supplements discussed below.

Among the supplements with the best scientific evidence for direct modulation of cortisol levels during periods of high stress are phosphatidylserine, beta-sitosterol, magnolia bark, and theanine. These four natural compounds are your most effective choices (your "best bets") for cortisol control. Choose one or more, either in consultation with a nutritional expert knowledgeable about supplements or after researching each one. (See the next section and Appendix B for more about how to choose and use supplements.) In crafting your own personal cortisol-control regimen, it may be helpful to refer to the table on page 35.

Dietary Supplements to Control Cortisol Levels

Supplement	Benefits	Drawbacks	Recommended daily dosage
Magnolia bark	Controls cortisol and has general effects as an antianxiety and anti-stress agent	Too much could cause sedation and drowsiness	200–800 mg
Beta-sitosterol	Balances ratio of cortisol to DHEA (one of the sex hormones), especially following the stress of exercise	None	30–300 mg
Theanine	Modulates brain waves for optimal physical and mental performance during stressful events	None	25–250 mg
Phosphatidylserine	Has a direct cortisol-lowering effect, especially after intense exercise	High cost at effective doses	50–100 mg

CHOOSING AND USING
SUPPLEMENTS WISELY

When choosing and using dietary supplements—particularly herbal supplements—it is important to exercise caution and to respect dosage recommendations. Here are a few basic considerations to keep in mind when selecting supplements to add to your daily regimen:

◆ Purchase supplements only from a reputable retailer that can provide you with a full disclosure of the ingredients, the manufacturing process, usage recommendations, and scientific evidence of safety and effectiveness.

◆ Respect the dosage and usage recommendations given by the manufacturer as you would for any prescription or over-the-counter medication. Herbal supplements, while "natural," are still medicinal in nature and should be considered natural medicines. Avoid falling into the trap of thinking that a higher dosage of a particular herbal will necessarily work any better or faster than the recommended dose.

◆ If you are taking any other supplements or medicines (especially prescription meds), consult with a knowledgeable expert on dietary supplements before embarking on any supplement regimen. Always discuss your use of any and all dietary supplements with your primary health-care provider—this is especially important if you are considering any medical or surgical procedures.

Chapter Highlights

◆ Controlling stress and thus minimizing cortisol exposure is the first and foremost factor influencing healthy and successful weight loss and long life.

◆ Stress makes us fat primarily because cortisol generally stimulates the overall appetite and also specifically triggers cravings for sweets and fats ("comfort" foods).

◆ Cortisol also sends a potent signal to abdominal fat cells (those in your belly region) to store as much fat as possible—and hold on to it.

◆ Any form of stress—whether physical, environmental, or psychological (even dieting!)—can increase cortisol levels and lead to weight gain.

◆ Follow any or all aspects of the SENSE program (stress management, exercise, nutrition, supplementation, and evaluation) to control cortisol levels.

◆ The Cortisol Connection Diet incorporates the most effective cortisol-controlling guidelines in the realms of exercise, nutrition, and supplementation and uses them to focus your metabolism toward weight loss.

◆ Supplements for cortisol control include a daily balanced multivitamin (B-complex, vitamin C, magnesium, and calcium), plus specialized herbals such as magnolia bark, theanine, beta-sitosterol, and phosphatidylserine.

Dennise

I can't believe the results from Dr. Talbott's Cortisol Connection program—and I almost feel as if I don't deserve them because they came so easily. My results have been terrific, with a loss of 8 percent body fat and almost twenty pounds. But the best part is that the balance in the plan between exercise and diet and supplements is something I can continue to follow forever. I appreciated Dr. Talbott's explaining the science behind the approaches in his program. Now I understand how these miraculous changes are happening in my body (the metabolism of it all). My husband is thrilled with the results— except for one small detail: None of my clothes fit anymore, which means shopping for a new wardrobe is in order (not that I will mind buying smaller sizes). Many thanks to Dr. Talbott and his staff for providing information that I could really use to help me have a more healthy and positive life.

CHAPTER 3

Blood-Sugar Control

Why control blood-sugar levels? Because keeping blood sugar within the proper range—versus allowing it to rise too high or drop too low—will dramatically enhance both fat burning and appetite control. Whenever blood sugar rises too high or falls too low, the body is signaled to stop burning fat. In the "too high" scenario, fat-burning stops because you have all that sugar in your system—the body decides to either burn or store the incoming sugar and save its stored fat for later use. In the "too low" scenario, the body stops burning fat because it lacks enough glucose to "prime" your metabolic fat-burning engine. This is because certain breakdown products from carbohydrate metabolism are needed to get fat metabolism going and keep it going. In addition, the "too low" scenario sets off alarm bells in the brain (which relies on glucose as its primary fuel source), and the brain responds with its own set of signals that increase your appetite—especially for more carbohydrates.

LOW-CARB VERSUS LOW-FAT: WHAT TO EAT?

Although scientific studies show us that low-fat/high-carbo-hydrate diets can certainly help you lose weight, they can be difficult to follow because of the problems associated with selecting the "right" kinds of carbohydrates at every single meal. When you eat the "wrong" type of carbohydrate-rich meal, your blood-sugar and insulin levels spike and then quickly drop, which can make you crave even more carbohydrates soon after eating. High blood-sugar levels and chronically high insulin levels can also lead to increased fat storage and reduced rates of fat breakdown (more on that topic appears in the following section).

At the other end of the spectrum, many of the popular *low*-carbohydrate diets do a decent job of taking care of the blood-sugar-control aspects of weight-loss metabolism, but they can also elevate cortisol levels—so the overall effect for most people is rapid weight loss (during the first few weeks of the diet), followed by a plateau, and then by a slow weight regain over a period of several months. Indeed, two very recent studies, published in *The New England Journal of Medicine* in 2003, showed that although early weight loss (during the first three months) on a low-carbohydrate diet is greater than on a low-fat diet, total weight loss after one year was comparable between the two dietary approaches. Similar studies of very low-fat Hawaiian diets and moderate-fat Mediterranean diets have shown similar magnitudes of weight loss and duration of weight maintenance.

WHY DIETS WORK

Virtually any diet will help you lose weight—at least for a period of time. I am always baffled by the number of people who ask me which diet is "best"—to which I reply, "None of them, and all of them" (a baffling question deserves a baffling answer). The point here is that your "diet personality" might have as much (or more) to do with your likelihood for success as the particular diet you choose. For example, the reason that many popular diets "fail" is not due to the diet being a poor diet, nor is the failure due to the dieter being a weak person, but rather it is due to a mismatch between the diet and the dieter. Very much like matching the fuel to the engine (gas in a gasoline engine and diesel in a diesel engine), the importance of matching the diet (low-carb, or low-fat, or balanced) to the dieter cannot be overemphasized. Across all the various permutations of matching diet and dieter (a topic for another book), however, there is a common thread: Diets that are more restrictive and result in greater feelings of deprivation tend to be the same diets that offer the worst long-term success rates.

For example, at the American Heart Association Annual Scientific Meeting in 2003, researchers from Tufts University presented a study in which four popular diet plans were compared. The study involved 160 overweight subjects with an average weight of 220 pounds and with 30 to 80 pounds to lose. The subjects were divided into four groups of 40. Each group followed either the Atkins diet (low carb/high fat), the Ornish diet (very low fat), the Zone diet (calories from 40 percent carbs/30 percent protein/30 percent fat), or Weight Watchers (moderate fat/carb/protein). After following the diets for one year, it was clear that each diet was equally effective in inducing weight loss: All four resulted in 10 to 12 pounds of weight loss over twelve months (not exactly spectacular results). More telling, however, was the fact that after only two months on the diets, 22 percent of the subjects had given up and dropped out of the study. At the one-year mark, more than half of the subjects had dropped out of the most restrictive Atkins (low-carb) and Ornish (low-fat) plans, while a full 35 percent had dropped out of the more balanced Zone and Weight Watchers programs. The conclusion we can draw from this study is that there is no "best" weight-loss diet—but there are clearly certain people who may be able to adhere to certain diets better than they can adhere to other types of diets (i.e., an individual's "diet personality"). Upon finding the "right" match between diet and dieter, the metabolic control points (MCPs) of cortisol, blood sugar, thermogenesis, thyroid hormones, serotonin, and norepinephrine can be brought together to optimize the weight-loss benefits of any diet. Imagine: Atkins could be better for carb counters, Ornish could be optimized for fat phobes, Zone could be more effective for 40/30/30-ers, and Weight Watchers could be enhanced for calorie (point) counters.

THE IMPACT OF INSULIN

Although a primary focal point of the Cortisol Connection Diet is the close relationship between stress, cortisol, and weight gain, a key intermediary in this relationship is another hormone called *insulin*.

Most people associate insulin problems with diabetes because of its primary role in regulating blood-sugar levels, but insulin has many additional functions in the body. Not only does insulin regulate blood-sugar levels within an extremely narrow range; it is also responsible for getting fat stored in our fat cells (adipose tissue), getting sugar stored in our liver and muscle cells (as glycogen), and getting amino acids directed toward protein synthesis (to build muscle). Due to these varied actions, insulin is sometimes thought of as a "storage hormone" because it helps the body put all of these great sources of energy away in their respective places for use later. Unfortunately, *storage* isn't exactly what we're after when we're trying to lose weight—so insulin is viewed (incorrectly) by many popular diets (and diet gurus) as "bad" because of its storage role.

Because insulin stimulates fat synthesis and promotes fat storage, there is a widespread belief that insulin circulating in the body induces weight gain. This misconception has led to a variety of diets that promote the idea that weight loss can be achieved by avoiding foods, such as carbohydrates, that stimulate insulin secretion. (Based on this line of thinking, the earlier discussion of the Tufts/AHA study should raise some questions about the claim that carbs are making you fat.) Unfortunately, this simplistic view of energy metabolism is only partly correct, and proponents of these diets fail to distinguish between a *normal* insulin response to meals (in which temporarily elevated blood levels of insulin quickly return to normal levels after meals) and an *abnormal* insulin metabolism (in which elevated insulin levels stay elevated for prolonged periods following meals).

With the Cortisol Connection Diet, levels of both insulin and leptin will *rise appropriately* following meals (which provides appetite-controlling benefits), but they will also *fall appropriately* (which provides the metabolic and thermogenic benefits needed to encourage weight loss and long-term weight maintenance).

The abnormal insulin metabolism referred to above— known as *insulin resistance*—leads to a reduction in the body's cellular response to insulin, which interferes with regulation of blood sugar, increases appetite, and blocks the body's ability to burn fat. When insulin resistance is combined with a poor diet (high in fat and/or refined carbohydrates), the result is the metabolic condition known as *syndrome X*, a disorder that can have an impact on virtually every disease process in the body.

Some authors have proposed that both insulin resistance and syndrome X are caused by a diet high in refined carbohydrates, such as those found in cookies, soft drinks, pasta, cereals, muffins, breads, rolls, and the like. While it is indeed true that refined carbohydrates can raise blood levels of glucose and insulin, it is not exactly true that they *cause* syndrome X. What is more likely is that the metabolic cascade of events set in motion by cortisol, and its interference with insulin function, is the primary factor in getting a person started toward developing full-blown syndrome X—and a poor diet tends to hasten the trip.

THE LINK BETWEEN CORTISOL AND BLOOD SUGAR

Having said all that, the bottom line for weight loss appears to be that controlling your cortisol levels is important at *all* times, while a targeted control of blood-sugar levels is most important at *specific* times—those times being the few hours following each meal. Eating a low-balance-factor meal (high in refined carbohydrates and not balanced with protein, fat, and fiber) tends to leave most people with low energy levels and "fuzzy" mental functioning. People who eat this type of diet for more than a few days will also notice that their clothes begin to fit a bit tighter due to a gradual weight gain of a pound or so at a time, especially around the mid-section. Soon they will begin to notice that they have trouble losing those extra few pounds. Taken separately, each of these relatively mild changes in one's metabolic machinery is not a big deal and is likely to be brushed off with an overly simplistic resolution to "get more exercise" or "watch what I eat."

By contrast, when you craft and consume meals based on the balance-factor/helping-hand approach, your blood-sugar response to each meal will be greatly modulated, and you'll feel the difference in your energy levels, mental concentration, and eventually in how your clothes fit and how you look.

Adding to the connection between cortisol and insulin resistance is the recent finding that inadequate sleep may actually cause insulin resistance. This is particularly interesting because of the well-known link between sleep deprivation and elevated cortisol levels. In 2001, at the Annual Scientific Meeting of the American Diabetes Association, sleep researchers from the University of Chicago showed that inadequate sleep leads to increased cortisol levels, insulin resistance, higher blood-sugar levels, elevated appetite, and weight gain. The research team compared "normal" sleepers (averaging 7.5 to 8.5 hours of sleep per night) to "short" sleepers (averaging less than 6.5 hours of sleep per night). They found that the "short" sleepers secreted 50 percent more cortisol and insulin, and were 40 percent less sensitive to the effects of insulin, than the "normal" sleepers. The researchers also suggested that sleep deprivation may play a significant role in the current epidemic of obesity and type-2 diabetes. Add to this the results from a recent poll conducted by the National Sleep Foundation, which found a steady decline in the number of hours that Americans sleep each night. In 1910, the average American slept a whopping 9 hours per night. In 1975, it was down to about 7.5 hours. Today, we average only about 7 hours of sleep per night—and many of us get far less than that.

The bottom line with blood-sugar control is that you can easily take the following three extremely important steps to improve your insulin sensitivity and your overall blood-sugar control:

1. Get some sleep (at least 7.5 hours per day if you can).

2. Control your cortisol levels (to improve insulin sensitivity).

3. Eat balanced meals according to the balance-factor approach (to slow the rise in blood sugar following meals).

Lisa

I work more than fifty hours each week, and on top of that I teach college classes and stay active in the community and my church. So it's easy to see that I don't really have an "off" switch. I've always wondered with all my activity why I have always had such trouble losing weight—but little did I know that stress has been playing such a large role in sabotaging my efforts.

Amazingly, I think Dr. Talbott's program and the information I learned is what pulled me through this rather insanely hectic time over the past several months. The idea of managing my cortisol helped me understand I was in control instead of life controlling me. Of course I realize there has to be balance in one's life, yet simply changing eating patterns and following Dr. Talbott's balance-factor and helping-hand approach (what I eat and when I eat it) has enabled me to feel satiated and brings calmness to my life.

I've done all the popular diets and group programs out there—and sometimes they work for awhile but never offer a long-term solution that works for me. When I heard about Dr. Talbott's program, it made a lot of sense (especially the SENSE part that combines stress control with diet and exercise). Most importantly, I am back to enjoying food again, because I don't have to worry about finding the "right" food or avoiding the "banned" foods when traveling for work. I now feel savvy enough about how food affects my metabolism and I know how to balance things out—for the first time ever I feel like I can eat without being afraid of gaining weight. And you know what makes that great? I'm losing fat and fitting into smaller clothes while I'm doing it—and who would have ever guessed?

Lastly, this entire Cortisol Connection Diet has been built into my lifestyle very easily—even with my crazy, busy, over-the-top, no-time lifestyle. Since starting Dr. Talbott's program I have been sharing the experiences and advice with all of my coworkers and everyone is following along with tremendous results. We've got the religion and we have Dr. Talbott to thank!

THE GLYCEMIC INDEX: DEFINING GOOD AND BAD CARBOHYDRATES

Lab researchers have assigned many foods with a rating known as the *glycemic index* (GI), which refers to the degree by which the food increases blood-sugar levels. For example, white bread has a GI of 69, and grapefruit has a GI of 26 (but not everyone agrees on the GI of every food; more on that issue below). A food with a high GI will rapidly increase blood-sugar levels, while a food with a low GI will have a less pronounced effect on blood-sugar levels. There is no doubt that the glycemic index has helped nutrition researchers gain a greater understanding of the metabolic and health properties associated with many foods. For example, several good studies show that long-term consumption of a diet with a high *glycemic load* (GL, which is an index of GI and total carbohydrate content of the diet) is a significant predictor of weight gain as well as of risk for diabetes and cardiovascular disease. Unfortunately, both the GI and the GL represent only part of a very complicated metabolic story—and using the GI or GL of specific foods to guide you in your weight-loss efforts is problematic for several reasons, some of which are explained below.

For one, the GI assigned to any given food is based on the blood-sugar response of six to twelve healthy subjects to a test meal of 50 grams of carbohydrate from that food—and that response is compared to their blood-sugar response to 50 grams of pure glucose. The GL gives a better picture of the real effects of eating a serving of a particular food because it also considers the total carbohydrate content of the food. But both the GI and the GL are misleading because they are calculated for isolated foods—and nobody is (or should be) sitting down to a meal composed solely of white bread, puffed rice, or plain macaroni (all foods with a high GI and therefore "banned" by some popular diets).

From a purely practical point of view, even trying to determine the GI or GL value of a particular food is nearly impossible outside of a metabolic lab. For example, something as simple and apparently straightforward as rice shows a huge range of measured GI values—which may be due to the different varieties of rice that are available (long grain versus short grain, etc.), their fiber content (white versus brown), and even the cooking method used to prepare the rice. Another example is carrots, which published GI values place into either a "high" GI category of 92 or a "low" GI category of 32. In addition, the GI and GL values of particular foods are significantly affected by factors that have nothing to do with the actual food—such as cooking methods (longer cooking tends to increase the GI of pasta, rice, and other foods); processing levels (smaller particle sizes tend to increase the GI of flours and other grains); and the content of fiber, fat, and protein contained in the overall meal (higher levels of each of these components tend to reduce the GI).

Many other factors can significantly influence the GI or GL of a particular food, including:

◆ the ripeness of fruit (riper = a lower GI)

◆ the physical form of the food (applesauce has a 25 percent higher GI than whole apple)

◆ the proportion of different carbohydrate types in a single food (such as rice, which can have different levels of

amylose, a slowly digested carb, versus amylopectin, a
rapidly digested carb)

◆ the shape of the food (such as different forms of pasta,
which can range from a GI value of 68 for macaroni to
45 for spaghetti; even thick linguine has a GI of 68,
while thin linguini scores a GI of 87)

◆ processing methods (foods that are "more" processed
tend to increase blood-sugar levels faster than those that
are "less" processed, but it is exceedingly difficult to
know the processes of grinding, rolling, and pressing that
your cake mix underwent before it arrived on your gro-
cer's shelf)

◆ preparation methods (including the amount of heat and
water used in cooking, the time of cooking, and even
the sizes into which the food particles are chopped
prior to cooking)

The problems with the GI have led many dieticians and
nutritionists to simplify their recommendations by educating
their clients to eat "complex" carbohydrates (starches)
instead of "simple" ones (sugars). But this approach does not
necessarily ensure consumption of the right foods. For example, white bread, mashed potatoes, and chocolate cake would
be a poor example of a meal consisting of "complex" carbohydrates. In general terms, refined-grain products ("complex"
or not) and potatoes tend to rapidly increase blood-sugar levels—unless they are combined with appropriate amounts of
protein, fat, and fiber (as they would be in a high-balance-
factor meal). Nuts, beans, legumes, and minimally processed
("whole") grains tend to have only a moderate effect on
blood-sugar levels, and most fruits and vegetables have a
small effect on blood-sugar levels, but even these foods still

need to be combined with appropriate metabolic regulators in the form of added protein or fat for optimal weight-loss results.

If these weren't already enough reasons to abandon the glycemic index as a practical method for achieving lasting weight loss, there is also the fact that for every study showing that a low-GI diet induces weight loss, another exists showing that a high-GI diet induces just as much weight loss with just as much satiety. For these and other reasons, the American Diabetes Association, the American Heart Association, and the American Dietetics Association do not recommend using GI values for dietary counseling.

That said, the Cortisol Connection Diet incorporates some important aspects of the glycemic index, such as encouraging the consumption of "whole" grains over highly refined ones. However, the Cortisol Connection Diet is also more practical to use as a day-in and day-out approach to weight loss because it balances blood-sugar levels (as a GI-based approach would do) and also balances cortisol levels, increases thermogenesis, helps to control portion sizes and overall calorie intake—and is easy to follow at the same time.

DIETARY SUPPLEMENTS FOR BLOOD-SUGAR CONTROL

Remember that optimal control of blood sugar is closely related to reducing a person's risk for diabetes, heart disease, syndrome X, and, of course, weight gain. Controlling blood-sugar levels also helps to control appetite. Luckily, many of our blood-sugar-control needs will be addressed by our eating patterns on the Cortisol Connection Diet and our daily intake of a comprehensive multivitamin/multimineral supplement. Of primary importance for blood-sugar control are the trace minerals chromium and vanadium, both of which are involved with the actions of insulin in regulating blood-sugar levels. Secondarily—but perhaps just as important for people who need additional blood-sugar control at meals—is an Indian herb known as banaba leaf. For a summary of information on dietary supplements that help control blood-sugar levels, see the table on page 53.

Chromium

Chromium is an essential trace mineral that aids in glucose metabolism, insulin regulation, and appetite control. A deficiency of chromium is known to lead to glucose intolerance and insulin resistance—which we know can predispose us to weight gain. In overweight individuals, chromium supplements of 200–400 mcg (micrograms) per day have been shown to improve glucose tolerance, normalize insulin levels, and help subjects lose about 50 percent more fat in three months than a placebo group. These results are probably due to the mineral's direct effect on controlling blood-sugar levels and modulating appetite and cravings.

Vanadium

Vanadium is another trace element involved in promoting normal insulin function. Safe and adequate dietary intakes fall within the range of approximately 10–100 mcg/day. Vanadium is thought to mimic the physiological effects of insulin and thereby to maintain blood-glucose levels, control appetite, and stimulate protein synthesis for muscle growth. Unfortunately, vanadium is one of the essential trace minerals that is often lacking in many multivitamin/mineral supplements, so be sure to check the label of any multi that you're considering purchasing. At the recommended doses (10–100 mcg/day), vanadium is considered quite safe, but some bodybuilding supplements are known to contain vanadium at potentially toxic milligram levels (about one thousand times higher than the amounts needed for blood-sugar control).

Banaba Leaf

Banaba leaf (*Lagerstroemia speciosa*) is a medicinal plant that grows in India, Southeast Asia, and the Philippines. Traditional uses include brewing tea from the leaves as a treatment for diabetes and hyperglycemia (elevated blood sugar). The blood-sugar-lowering effect of banaba-leaf extract is similar to that of insulin, which improves glucose transport from the blood into body cells. The blood-sugar-regulating properties of banaba have been demonstrated in studies of isolated cells, both animal and human. In isolated cells, one of the active compounds in banaba extract, corosolic acid, is known to stimulate glucose uptake. In diabetic mice, rats, and rabbits, banaba consumption reduces elevated blood-sugar and insulin levels to normal. In humans with type-2 diabetes, 16–48 mg/day of banaba extract, taken for four to eight weeks, has been shown to reduce blood-sugar levels by 5–30 percent and to help subjects maintain a tighter control of blood-sugar fluctuations. An interesting side effect of the tighter blood-sugar control in these studies is a tendency of banaba to control appetite and promote weight loss—an average of two to four pounds per month—without significant dietary alterations.

Chapter Highlights

◆ The Cortisol Connection Diet controls not only cortisol levels but also blood-sugar levels. It is important to understand that the combined metabolic effects of modulating cortisol and blood-sugar levels simultane-

Dietary Supplements to Control Blood-Sugar Levels

Supplement	Benefits	Cautions	Recommended daily dosage
Chromium	Works with insulin to control blood-sugar levels	None	100–400 mcg
Vanadium	Works with insulin to control blood-sugar levels	None	10–100 mcg
Banaba (Lagerstroemia speciosa)	Modulates the rise in blood-sugar levels following meals. Controls appetite and reduces body weight	Diabetics may need to reduce medications for blood-sugar control	10–100 mg

ously can mean the difference between weight-loss success or failure for many people.

◆ Poor blood-sugar control reduces fat burning and increases appetite. Optimal blood-sugar control increases fat burning and reduces appetite.

◆ Low-fat and low-carb diets can induce weight loss, but when either type of diet becomes too restrictive, cortisol levels become elevated and the diet loses effectiveness.

◆ Carbohydrates and insulin will not make you fat, but you want blood-sugar and insulin levels to rise appropriately and fall appropriately following a meal for optimal control of appetite and energy metabolism.

- Cortisol (from stress) will interfere with insulin function and thus with blood-sugar levels.

- Don't worry about the complexities of the glycemic index (GI) or glycemic load (GL). Instead, focus on using the balance factor combined with the helping hand approach to control blood-sugar response at each meal.

- Get enough sleep. As little as one hour of lost sleep can increase cortisol levels by 50 percent and interfere with insulin function.

- Dietary supplements for daily blood-sugar control include chromium, vanadium, and banaba-leaf extract.

Laura

I'm not sure where to begin in telling of the benefits I have achieved with Dr. Talbott's Cortisol Connection Diet. I came into the program not for weight loss (though that was an added side benefit), but rather for health reasons. I was diagnosed with diabetes a few months before trying Dr. Talbott's program, and my main interest was finding something that would help me control my diabetes. The fact that the program focused partly on controlling blood sugar made it seem like a good thing to try—but I never expected all the wonderful benefits in how I look and feel. By following Dr. Talbott's program, I lost more than five inches off my waist and have gone from a size 22 to a size 16. Plus, my friends tell me that I look happier, and I can certainly tell that my stress level is down.

The program is so easy to follow that I never really felt I was on any kind of a "diet." But I certainly have the results to show for it. The most noticeable part of Dr. Talbott's program for me was that right away I noticed it helped to stop my cravings for carbs and sugar. After the program, my doctor was amazed that the results of my A1C test (how high my blood sugar was during Dr. Talbott's three-month program) had been cut in half—and my doctor couldn't believe how fast and how far it had come down. I am pleased that Dr. Talbott has created such an easy-to-follow program that makes sense and is able to help so many people, including me.

. . . .
.
.

CHAPTER 4

Thermogenesis

The term thermogenesis refers to the generation of heat (thermo- means "heat"; -genesis means "create"). In the body, heat creation comes from the conversion of food into energy: Heat is given off as a by-product of energy metabolism. Some people are simply born with highly effective thermogenesis mechanisms, so they are able to shed excess weight or maintain their ideal weight without too much effort. You know who they are—the folks who seem to eat whatever they want and never gain an ounce.

The millions of other people who need to burn more calories than they are burning right now can increase their level of thermogenesis in several ways—such as by eating more, eating more of the right foods, and exercising. Simply eating more food tends to increase thermogenesis up to a point, but then the inevitable happens: You start to gain weight because you don't burn off as many calories as you take in. A better approach is to eat more of the right foods—and an even better approach is to eat those right foods in the right combinations to boost thermogenesis even more. By following the balance-factor and helping-hand approaches outlined in Chapter 1, you'll achieve the optimal combination of thermogenic macronutrients.

WE'RE NOT GETTING ANY YOUNGER

As we age, our metabolic rate drops, and most of us begin to pack on the pounds. If, in response to stress, we add that fat to our abdominal area, our body changes shape from that of an hourglass to one more resembling a shot glass—and repeated diets only compound the problem.

Most of us will experience a drop in metabolism of about 0.5 percent per year after the age of twenty (see table below). This phenomenon is largely due to a loss of about five to ten pounds of muscle tissue every decade. Half a percentage point may seem like a small decrease, but when we consider the effects over ten or twenty years, it means that we're burning 5 percent fewer calories at age thirty and 10 percent fewer calories at age forty—and so it goes, with about 5 percent fewer calories burned for every ten years of age. Just imagine: By the time we turn fifty, we're burning 15 percent fewer calories than we did when we were twenty.

Change in Metabolic Rate and Weight Gain with Age

Age (years)	Calorie needs (daily)	Drop in daily metabolic rate (from age 20)	Pounds of extra fat (from age 20)*
20	2,000–2,500	—	—
30	1,900–2,375	100–125 calories	10
40	1,800–2,250	200–250 calories	20
50	1,700–2,125	300–375 calories	30
60	1,600–2,000	400–500 calories	40
70	1,500–1,875	500–625 calories	50

* without a corresponding change in diet/exercise patterns

How does this translate into a way to maintain your youthful figure? An average-size person, consuming about 2,000 calories per day at age twenty, needs only 1,700 calories at age fifty to maintain his or her body weight. That's 300 fewer calories per day. This means that if you don't make some serious changes in your diet and exercise patterns, your fifty-year-old body will be carrying around thirty extra pounds of fat compared to when you were twenty!

Connie

Coming into Dr. Talbott's program I felt I was ready for a change in my lifestyle in order to become a "healthy" person. I had already made a commitment to myself at the beginning of the new year to try to make changes in my diet and exercise programs. This program came at the right time and made all the difference for me because I had read and tried just about every diet out there and had decided that I needed to do something different. Dr. Talbott's program seemed to combine all the best aspects of the other diets without any of the silly gimmicks. But the best part was that it was so balanced and simple to follow that it easily became part of the healthy lifestyle that I had been searching for.

I really didn't set high goals for myself at the beginning. I only wanted to work on a more healthy diet and to stop gaining so much weight. If I could get some weight loss along with a healthier lifestyle, then that would be an added bonus. I found the nutritional information and the education about metabolism that Dr. Talbott gave us to be invaluable and on the cutting edge. I've been reading a lot about nutrition and how the body responds to emotions, so I understand the "Cortisol Connection" that Dr. Talbott talks about and how important it is. The connections between emotions and how our bodies work is real, and now I am living proof.

I am quite surprised and thrilled at the results after twelve weeks on Dr. Talbott's program. I've lost weight and inches—all without really "trying" to do anything but slow/stop my weight gain, and even with about three weeks of vacation and indulging in all kinds of delicious foods. The program has helped me change my attitude about food. I am making better choices to match the balance of nutrients that Dr. Talbott talks about in his program. I am now sharing my experiences with my friends, family, and neighbors because I know that if Dr. Talbott's program can help me to work towards a better me, then it can help anybody.

ENHANCING THERMOGENESIS

The most dramatic increases in thermogenesis will come from a diet that controls cortisol and blood-sugar levels within their normal ranges (as the Cortisol Connection Diet does) and provides a balanced intake of all the macronutrients, that is, of protein, carbohydrate, and fat (as the Cortisol Connection Diet also does). Good scientific data show us that higher levels of thermogenesis are associated with lower levels of body fat, and that people with higher levels of thermogenesis are less likely to store energy as body fat. These "high-thermogenic" people are "hot" in at least a couple of ways: They burn more calories (which creates more heat), and they carry less body fat (so they look good and feel great).

So, what do these high-thermogenic people eat? They eat a balanced diet that provides approximately 1,300–1,800 calories per day. Calories only come from carbohydrates (4 calories per gram), protein (4 calories per gram), and fat (9 calories per gram)—and also from alcohol (7 calories per gram). And these high-thermogenic folks tend to consume macronutrients in roughly the following ratios:

- ◆ Carbohydrates: about 200 grams/day, primarily from whole grains, fruits, and vegetables;

- ◆ Protein: about 70 grams/day, primarily from lean sources such as chicken and fish;

- ◆ Fat: about 40 grams/day, primarily from seeds, nuts, olive oil, and canola oil.

If you do the math, these folks are eating a diet that provides calories in a ratio of about 55 percent from carbohydrate, 20 percent from protein, and 25 percent from fat—or exactly the proportions that you would automatically get if you were following the Cortisol Connection approach to eating. If you followed these people for several years, as researchers at the National Weight Control Registry at the University of Colorado Health Sciences Center have done, you'd see that not only have they lost an average of sixty-six pounds, they have kept it off for more than five years! When it comes to sheer magnitude of weight loss and duration of weight maintenance, no other dietary approach even comes close to matching these numbers.

Many people attempt to eat "right" and follow a regular exercise program, and yet they still seem to gain weight. One of the reasons may be a change in their thermogenic potential (their ability to burn sufficient calories) because of some small (but important) dietary choices. Researchers at the University of Massachusetts have shown, for example, that certain dietary patterns, such as eating one or more midday snacks, are associated with a reduced risk of obesity (39 percent reduction in the case of healthy snacking), while other dietary habits, such as skipping breakfast, can increase obesity risk (450 percent increase in obesity risk from skipping breakfast). The dramatic difference here is largely due to a change in metabolic rate (snacking increases it, while skipping breakfast reduces it)—so dietary patterns that encourage a greater expenditure of calories are also those that tend to result in a lower body weight over time. In the case of breakfast, even our grandmothers told us that it is the "most important meal of the day," but when it comes to dieting you should consider breakfast a "free" meal! This is because eating breakfast increases your metabolic rate by 100–200 calories—while skipping breakfast slows down your metabolism by about the same amount. This means that by skipping breakfast (when compared to eating it), the overall difference balances out at 200–400 calories of lost calorie burning (thus the whopping 450 percent increase in obesity risk noted by the University of Massachusetts researchers).

Before we continue with our discussion of ways to enhance thermogenesis, let's consider a few guidelines that everyone who's attempting to lose weight should be aware of.

Caution: Calorie restriction will reduce your overall metabolic rate.

Acute calorie restriction typically causes a sharp decline in body temperature and the number of calories that you'll burn in a given day. By spacing high-balance-factor meals and snacks throughout the day, and eating them in the right proportions (hand, fist, palm, etc.), you'll balance calorie levels to counteract this drop in metabolic rate.

In addition, most of us can also benefit from directly boosting thermogenesis to help our bodies burn even more calories throughout the day. Fortunately, certain dietary supplements, including calcium and green tea, can be a safe and effective way to help increase our metabolic rate (see the section "Dietary Supplements to Enhance Thermogenesis" starting on page 65).

Caution: Dehydration—lack of water—will reduce your thermogenic potential.

Drink plenty of water! Water is an important catalyst for weight loss because proper hydration is essential for fat burning, maintenance of muscle mass, and boosting overall metabolism. If you're dehydrated, even to a slight degree, your cortisol levels will rise and your metabolic rate will drop. Your hydration needs vary based on environmental conditions and exercise levels, but the rule of thumb to drink eight glasses of water a day is a good one. It's based on a chemical estimate of how much water is needed to metabolize 1,500–2,000 calories derived from a mixed diet.

Caution: Boosting thermogenesis will increase free-radical production.

As your body converts nutrients into energy, it creates toxic molecules called *free radicals*, which can damage cellular structures, DNA, and delicate tissues, such as eyes, lungs, and blood vessels. Over time, this microscopic free-radical damage will wear down tissues and organs and lead to premature aging. The good news is that a large proportion of free-radical damage can be prevented by dietary antioxidants.

Additional levels of dietary antioxidants are always a good idea to include in any regimen that boosts thermogenesis (which, again, increases caloric expenditure, but also increases the generation of free radicals). In addition, in our modern world that is filled with highly processed foods, we need to be aware that any foods that rapidly increase blood-glucose levels will cause a direct fall in blood levels of antioxidants, even when they are balanced with appropriate foods into a high-balance-factor meal.

Antioxidants include nutrients you've heard of, such as vitamins C and E, as well as some that are probably less familiar to you, such as thiols (selenium, cysteine, alpha-lipoic acid), carotenoids (beta-carotene, lutein, lycopene), and flavonoids (catechins, polyphenols, isoflavones). Brightly colored fruits and vegetables are the richest sources of these antioxidants. Unfortunately, although the American Cancer Society and most worldwide health organizations recommend that we consume five to ten servings of fruits and vegetables per day to get enough antioxidants, nearly 90 percent of American adults (and 98 percent of children) fail to do so. Therefore, a daily antioxidant supplement is important for everyone—but it's vital for anybody following a thermogenic regimen (in order to counteract the increased free-radical damage). An antioxidant supplement needs to be balanced to supply representatives of each part of the antioxidant network. So when you're shopping for an antioxidant supplement, be sure to look for one that provides balanced levels of vitamin C, vitamin E, thiols, carotenoids, and flavonoids—and not simply a whopping dose of any single antioxidant.

WEIGHT-LOSS SUPPLEMENTS TO AVOID

Among dietary supplements, those targeted to weight loss and weight maintenance represent the largest category in the entire supplement industry. The key problem, however, is that many of the most popular dietary supplements on the market can actually increase cortisol levels in the body and make long-term weight control more difficult. Even though many of them can be quite effective in suppressing appetite and increasing energy expenditure for a few weeks, these stimulants can also cause stress at the tissue and cellular levels. The body perceives this stimulant-mediated stress in the very same way that it perceives other forms of stress, and it responds by increasing the body's secretion of cortisol—which effectively sabotages any weight-loss success experienced in the first few weeks of use.

Using supplements of this type may help you lose weight during the early stages of weight loss, but they'll actually hurt your chances of long-term weight maintenance because of their effect of increasing cortisol levels. Among the most important supplements to avoid are the herbal stimulants ma huang (ephedra), *Sida cordifolia* (ephedra), guarana (caffeine), *Coleus forskolin*, and yohimbe (yohimbine), each of which will increase the output of adrenaline and cortisol from the adrenal glands.

The widespread popularity of the herbal stimulants, most notably ephedra, is due largely to the fact that they work—at least temporarily. Ephedra and related supplements are well known to kill a person's appetite and increase her or his energy levels, so over the course of a month or two that person will drop a few extra pounds. The downside, however, is the fact that while the short-term effects of these compounds are beneficial for weight loss (because they result in reduced appetite and increased caloric expenditure), the longer-term increase in cortisol levels is detrimental for a person's continued weight-loss efforts.

If the cortisol-increasing side effects of these potent herbal stimulants weren't already bad enough, researchers from Lausanne University, in Switzerland, have shown that as little as two days of ephedra consumption at 40 mg/day reduced glucose uptake and oxidation by 25 percent. When subjects were under additional mental stress, glucose uptake and oxidation dropped by more than 50 percent! This means that ephedra supplements inhibit the body's ability to use glucose as an energy source, so blood-sugar levels climb, fat metabolism shuts off, and hunger comes raging back. Similar findings have been noted for forskolin (the active ingredient in *Coleus forskohlii*), yohimbine (the active ingredient in *Pausinystalia yohimbe*), and caffeine (the active ingredient in *Paullinia cupana*, also known as *guarana*). For example, around 200 milligrams of caffeine (about the amount contained in two cups of coffee and in a single dose of many weight-loss supplements) will increase blood levels of cortisol and blood sugar by 30 percent within one hour.

So what to do? The most prudent approach would be to completely avoid these herbal stimulants in favor of a more balanced approach to promoting weight loss, such as eating several small meals spaced throughout the day; getting a balanced intake of protein, carbs, fat, and fiber; and participating in regular aerobic exercise plus resistance training—exactly the plan advocated by the Cortisol Connection Diet. That said, millions of people are likely to keep using products that contain herbal stimulants anyway (despite the U.S. Food and Drug Administration's ban on ephedra sales in April 2004). If you *do* decide to use any of these herbal stimulants, please do so with extreme caution—and try to curb your use of them after a month or two.

At the very least, the cortisol- and blood-sugar-raising effects of herbal stimulants should be counteracted by combining their use with one of the cortisol-controlling supplements outlined in Chapter 2. This combination will lessen the adverse side effects associated with elevated cortisol levels, while still allowing you to benefit from the short-term appetite-control and thermogenic/fat-burning effects of the herbal stimulants.

DIETARY SUPPLEMENTS TO ENHANCE THERMOGENESIS

A number of additional supplements are known to increase thermogenesis in humans—and all are considered to be extremely safe for long-term use because they work with your body's existing metabolic machinery to slightly enhance calorie expenditure. A summary of information on dietary supplements that enhance thermogenesis is given in the table on page 71.

Calcium

Studies at Purdue University and the University of Tennessee have shown that a calcium intake of 1,000 mg/day versus an intake of 500 mg/day can result in a weight difference of as much as twenty pounds over the course of two years. Researchers from the University of Colorado have shown that higher calcium intakes are associated with a higher rate of caloric expenditure and fat metabolism. Metabolic studies at the University of Tennessee have shown that cellular calcium levels are related to the production of cortisol in human fat cells. In these studies, depriving fat cells of calcium led to a direct and rapid three- to six-fold increase in cortisol production. This research suggests that maintaining an optimal calcium intake may be an important mechanism for reducing cortisol production in fat cells and reducing the accumulation of belly fat seen in high-stress people. Scientists at Creighton University have suggested that because calcium intake is so closely related to body weight, increasing calcium intake to recommended levels (1,000–1,500 mg/day, based on age and gender) could reduce the prevalence of obesity in the population by 60–80 percent!

Perhaps the most effective approaches for increasing your calcium intake are to eat more dairy products and more leafy green vegetables, and to add a calcium supplement to your daily regimen (enough to bring your total daily intake up to 1,200–1,500 mg/day). In doing so, you'll reduce cortisol production, stimulate thermogenesis, and promote weight loss. Since the average daily calcium intake for Americans is in the 750 mg/day range, a daily calcium supplement of 500–750 mg is often appropriate.

Green Tea

When it comes to green tea, the story is almost too good to be true. Imagine a supplement that increases caloric expenditure, reduces fat absorption, and is perfectly safe (the only "side effects" being a reduced risk of cancer and a fuller bust line). Now *that* would be a blockbuster supplement! Well, not only is that supplement on the shelves right now; it has been there for decades and we just didn't know of its weight-loss benefits. It's green-tea extract.

Scientific evidence has been mounting to support the idea that the polyphenol/catechins found at high levels in green tea (and at lower levels in some other plants) may act on the sympathetic nervous system and adrenal glands to increase calorie expenditure and fat burning. An additional effect of green tea appears to be an inhibition of the fat-digesting enzymes (lipases) in the gut, suggesting a reduction in fat digestion and absorption.

Several well-controlled clinical trials have shown that green-tea extract can increase twenty-four-hour energy expenditure and fat oxidation. One of the studies, published in *The American Journal of Clinical Nutrition* in 1999, compared a daily dose of green-tea extract to caffeine alone and also to a placebo. Results showed that the green tea caused a significant (14 percent) increase in twenty-four-hour energy expenditure (subjects burned about 280 extra calories) and enhanced fat oxidation by 34 percent over the twenty-four-hour period. These effects were significantly greater than those seen in the group receiving only caffeine, indicating that green tea has thermogenic properties and promotes fat oxidation beyond that which can be explained solely by its caffeine content.

Other studies from different research groups in Holland and China have shown that green tea increases resting energy expenditure by 6–8 percent compared to a placebo group, and that green-tea catechins improve several metabolic aspects related to syndrome X, including a 12–54 percent reduction in glucose and insulin levels, and a 20–26 percent increase in insulin sensitivity.

You may be wondering why in the preceding section I suggest that you avoid supplements containing high levels of caffeine (because too much caffeine can increase cortisol levels) and then turn around in this section and encourage you to drink green tea (which contains caffeine). The answer is because green tea is unique in the plant world in that it contains "just enough" caffeine to induce thermogenesis—when, that is, the caffeine is combined with a special class of naturally occurring flavonoids called *catechins*, as it is in green tea. Furthermore, green tea also contains a unique cortisol-controlling amino acid called *theanine* that counteracts the cortisol-increasing tendency of caffeine.

When choosing how to add green tea to your daily regimen, you can certainly opt for dosing your green tea cup by cup (drinking it), but this approach tends to deliver a variable amount of theanine, caffeine, and catechins, based on the type and age of the tea leaves and the steeping time of your tea. A more targeted (and preferred) approach is to take green-tea extract in capsule form. There are numerous products available, so be sure to select one that matches the profile of extracts used in clinical weight-loss studies (that is, providing both catechins and caffeine in the same extract).

The "moral" of the green-tea story is simple: Green-tea extract can increase daily calorie expenditure, enhance fat metabolism, and reduce fat absorption. As an interesting side note, a handful of animal studies published in biochemistry journals over the past few years have suggested that green tea can also enhance the growth of mammary (breast) tissues. In one series of studies conducted at Shizuoka University in Japan, green tea was shown to have a growth-promoting effect on mammary-gland development. Could it be that green tea slims the waist while boosting the bust? We'll have to wait for human studies to confirm these animal findings, so stay tuned....

Synephrine

Synephrine is the main active compound found in the fruit of a plant called bitter orange, or *Citrus aurantium*. The fruit is also known as *zhi shi* in traditional Chinese medicine and as green orange, sour orange, and bitter orange in other parts of the world. Synephrine is chemically very similar to the ephedrine found in a number of weight-loss and energy supplements that contain ma huang (a similarity that has caused synephrine to be labeled as the "chemical kissing cousin" of the ephedrine in ephedra). But synephrine differs from ephedrine in that synephrine is considered a *semi-selective sympathomimetic* (because it targets some tissues such as fat more than it targets others such as the heart and brain) versus a *non-selective sympathomimetic* (like ephedra, which targets many tissues equally and thus often causes side effects). For example, although some high-dose ephedra-containing supplements have been associated with certain cardiovascular side effects such as elevated blood pressure and heart palpitations, researchers at Mercer University in Atlanta have shown that *Citrus aurantium* extract has no effect on hemodynamics such as heart rate and blood pressure because it targets fat tissue rather than heart tissue.

Although synephrine is a mild stimulant for thermogenesis, similar in some ways to caffeine and ephedrine, it is
thought to have less pronounced effects in terms of providing an energy boost, suppressing appetite, and increasing
metabolic rate and caloric expenditure. This means that
synephrine is not likely to "charge" you up the way caffeine
and ephedra might, but it can still deliver a generalized
metabolic effect that aids in fat metabolism and weight loss.

In traditional Chinese medicine, *zhi shi* is used to help
stimulate *qi* (pronounced chee, and defined as the body's
vital energy or life force)—but in order to maximize the
metabolic benefits of these extracts, total synephrine intake
should probably be kept to a range of 10–50 mg/day.

A recent study conducted on dogs suggests that the
synephrine and octopamine found in *Citrus aurantium*
extracts can increase metabolic rate in a specific type of fat
tissue known as brown adipose tissue (BAT). This effect
would be expected to increase fat loss in humans, except for
one small detail: Adult humans don't have any brown adipose tissue to speak of—yet this claim stands as one of the
most overhyped promises on the weight-loss scene.

Until very recently, synephrine-containing supplements
existed solely because there were some interesting theories
on how they *might* work to increase metabolic rate and promote significant weight loss. At this writing, there are now at
least two clinical studies showing that synephrine-containing
supplements help promote weight loss, and at least three
clinical studies showing enhanced thermogenesis (calorie
expenditure) from these supplements. There is a great deal
of research currently underway into the weight-loss benefits
of synephrine and supplements with related thermogenic
effects, leading researchers in the Department of Physiology
at Georgetown University to conclude that *"Citrus aurantium may be the best thermogenic substitute for ephedra."*

Dietary Supplements to Enhance Thermogenesis

Supplement	Benefits	Drawbacks	Recommended daily dosage
Calcium	Enhances thermogenesis and cortisol control at the level of the fat cell (especially in the abdominal area)	None	500–750 mg as a supplement (daily intake from foods and supplements should be 1,200–1,500 mg total)
Green-tea extract (Camellia sinensis)	Enhances thermogenesis via maintenance of cellular norepinephrine levels	None	200–750 mg of a green tea extract standardized for polyphenols/catechins
Bitter orange extract (Citrus aurantium)	Enhances thermogenesis and stimulates fat mobilization at the level of the fat cell	None	100–250 mg of bitter orange extract standardized for synephrine

Chapter Highlights

◆ Thermogenesis means to "create heat," a process that occurs through the conversion of food into energy in the body. Thermogenesis is an important aspect of successful weight loss.

◆ Enhancing thermogenesis can be achieved by eating the right foods and the right combinations of foods (using the balance-factor and helping-hand approaches outlined in Chapter 1).

- Eat breakfast, consume healthy snacks during the day, and avoid dehydration to maintain optimal thermogenesis and metabolic rates throughout the day.

- Elevated thermogenesis also means elevated free-radical production and thus potential damage to cellular structures, so be sure to eat a diet rich in brightly colored fruits and vegetables to provide antioxidant phytonutrients. Also consider a balanced antioxidant supplement to combat free-radical damage.

- Avoid stimulant-based (e.g., caffeine-based) weight-loss supplements because they can interfere with cortisol and blood-sugar metabolism. The short-term appetite suppression of the stimulants is offset by increased cortisol levels and long-term weight gain.

- Thermogenic supplements with the best evidence for safety and effectiveness include calcium and green-tea extract.

Suzette

Since I'm an executive in a large benefits company, a mother of four, a grandmother of six, and a community activist, stress is not an occasional challenge for me—it's a constant companion. It was exactly this high stress level and the impact it was having on my physical and emotional health that prompted me to start on Dr. Talbott's Cortisol Connection Diet program.

I was immediately impressed with Dr. Talbott's unique focus on lifestyle changes rather than promoting the typical "dieting" mentality. I appreciated the realistic approaches to diet and exercise that he offered, and I never felt like I was encouraged to diet; rather, I was encouraged to become better informed about what effects certain foods would have on my overall health and why.

I learned the synergistic combination of natural supplements, eating smarter, and exercise to help control all the various aspects of my metabolism. Over the course of the program, I lost inches and pounds from my body and I enjoyed the way the program made me feel. I had more energy and a better mental outlook, rather than feeling fatigue and hunger, as is often the case with other diets.

Most importantly, Dr. Talbott's program has helped me realize what works for me, and I have used that knowledge to make more effective and healthier choices in exercise, foods, and supplements. This change in lifestyle has enabled me to manage my stress more effectively, and, in turn, the stress control has enabled me to lose even more weight and has rekindled my enthusiasm for exercise and for being more active in general. I would highly recommend this program to any person who has experienced the same dieting frustrations that I have in the past and is looking for a unique and educated approach to improved health and fitness.

. . . .
:
:

CHAPTER 5

General Metabolic Support

I could list dozens and dozens of mediating factors that affect energy metabolism and weight loss, ranging from appetite signals, to neurotransmitters, to genetics, to name just a few. These are all things that we might be able to influence and that might provide a modest benefit for weight loss. However, the most promising metabolic factors involve controlling cortisol, blood sugar, and thermogenesis. These are the metabolic control points (MCPs) that will deliver the biggest bang for your buck; therefore, comprehensive programs that address each of them simultaneously will be the most successful in helping you achieve and maintain lasting weight loss.

That said, there are some promising peripheral areas in addition to the ones addressed so far in this book that may provide benefits. They include metabolic support of thyroid, serotonin, and norepinephrine. On their own, manipulation of any or all of these factors (without simultaneous control of cortisol, blood sugar, and thermogenesis) is unlikely to provide substantial weight-loss benefits. But when added to a comprehensive program, as is the case in the Cortisol Connection Diet, addressing these MCPs can provide the added "metabolic oomph" needed to nudge you off a weight-loss plateau and into that new pair of jeans.

The exercise and nutrition regimen for balancing metabolism of thyroid, serotonin, and norepinephrine is the very same as the one outlined throughout this book for balancing cortisol, blood sugar, and thermogenesis. Thus, the recommendations that follow are geared more towards specific vitamins, minerals, and herbs known to support these areas.

THYROID SUPPORT

Here's an understatement: Thyroid function is important. It's not just important for weight maintenance and energy levels (which are the primary reasons for trying to stimulate or restore thyroid function), but also for libido, mental function, reproductive health, skin condition, cardiovascular health—and the list goes on and on. Because of the complex nature of thyroid-hormone metabolism, it would be overly simplistic to recommend a single nutrient or herb for "boosting" thyroid function. The most effective approach to thyroid support is a multifaceted one that optimizes thyroid activity by supporting the following four processes:

1. thyroid hormone synthesis;

2. conversion of T4 (inactive thyroid hormone) to T3 (active hormone);

3. a normal stress response, because cortisol blocks many thyroid functions; and

4. stabilization of cell-membrane structure, the location where T4 is converted to T3.

The general idea is that by addressing these four different but related areas of thyroid function, the overall activity of the thyroid hormones is optimized. The thyroid gland—located in the neck, near the voice box—is a very complex tissue. Just ask anyone who has ever struggled with having too much or too little thyroid hormone (*hyperthyroidism* and *hypothyroidism*, respectively): It's a nightmare. When thyroid hormones are "off," you feel terrible. You experience a lack of energy, trouble concentrating, weight gain, increased appetite, dry skin and hair, and other symptoms. For that reason, keeping the thyroid gland "happy," so it produces the right levels of active and inactive thyroid hormones in the right amounts and at the right times, is a vitally important aspect of overall metabolism.

In response to a hormone called *TSH* (thyroid-stimulating hormone, released from the pituitary gland in the brain), the thyroid gland produces another hormone called *T4*, which is then converted in peripheral tissues into another, more active form of thyroid hormone called *T3*. The process by which T4 is converted to T3 is known as *deiodination*. If you have too little TSH, then your thyroid can't make enough T4 and it has nothing to convert into active T3. If you have plenty of T4, but some problem with the conversion process, then you're also lacking enough T3. For example, stress hormones such as cortisol can inhibit the conversion of T4 to T3, so you could have all the TSH and T4 in the world but still lack enough active T3 to maintain metabolism because of the cortisol "block" on thyroid-hormone conversion.

What are some nutritional supplements that can support the healthy functioning of all these processes? On the T4-synthesis side of things, iodine and bladderwrack (an iodine-rich algae) are often used as supporting nutrients. Iodine is an essential mineral for synthesis of thyroid hormone—so essential that iodine is sequestered in the thyroid gland so there is enough of it to combine with tyrosine (an amino acid) in the synthesis of T4. For the second step, improving the conversion of T4 to T3, the essential trace minerals selenium and zinc act as cofactors for the function of the enzyme needed in the conversion of T4 to active T3.

That enzyme is named 5'-*deiodinase*. Low vitamin E levels have also been linked to reduced T3 levels, an effect that may have to do with the role of vitamin E in stabilizing cellular membranes, where 5'-deiodinase is located.

Guggul (*Commiphora mukul*) is a traditional Ayurvedic medicine used for treating lethargy and suppressed libido. Its metabolic benefits stem from the herb's content of guggulsterones as stimulators of thyroid-hormone synthesis. Other traditional approaches to supporting thyroid-gland function and thyroid-hormone metabolism include the use of antistress adaptogenic herbs, such as rhodiola (*Rhodiola rosea*). Adaptogenic herbs are used in traditional Chinese and Ayurvedic medicine to alleviate the symptoms of many stress-related diseases. Rhodiola in particular is known for its unique nonstimulant benefits as an energetic (tonic) herb, an effect that is thought to be mediated via control of cortisol, thus removing the blocking effects of cortisol on thyroid function. For a summary of information on dietary supplements that provide added metabolic support for thyroid function, see the table on page 80.

SEROTONIN AND NOREPINEPHRINE: NATURAL APPETITE CONTROL

Controlling overall appetite has been one of the most promising—and one of the most disappointing—areas researched for weight control over the past several decades. The promise lies in the fact that there are literally hundreds of appetite-regulating hormones, peptides, and neurotransmitters that have been identified in the brain, in the intestinal tract, in the stomach, and in the fat tissue. Thus, there are many possible targets for attempting to control appetite. Unfortunately, almost as soon as a promising new appetite signal is identified and targeted (typically with a drug that blocks the effects of that signal), an even newer signal is identified that overrides the first signal. This means you have to shut off the first signal, and then the second, and then the third, and so on until you have no more appetite signals "getting through" to the brain to stimulate hunger.

The hundreds of overlapping appetite signals have made the pharmaceutical control of appetite a frustrating series of starts, stops, and dead ends. Despite the frustration associated with trying to sort out the myriad appetite signals, however, there is at least one constant in the appetite-control research: Chronic stress (and thus cortisol exposure) are consistent stimulators of appetite, especially for the fats and sweets we view as "comfort" foods. For example, in a 2001 article in the journal *Psychoneuroendocrinology*, researchers from Yale and the University of California at San Francisco (UCSF) described how cortisol, induced by psychological stress, was a potent regulator of both appetite and mood: Women with more cortisol ate more sweets and had a more negative mood. Over time, the researchers noted, these alterations could impact both weight and health.

In a related series of experiments published in the proceedings of the National Academy of Sciences in 2003 and in the journal *Endocrinology* in 2004, another group of researchers from UCSF and Rockefeller University showed how chronic stress and cortisol overexposure may be one of the most potent appetite signals and a primary cause of obesity in our modern societies around the world.

It is interesting to note how stress (via cortisol) is a potent regulator of both appetite and mood. The drug Meridia (sibutramine), one of the two existing pharmaceuticals for weight loss, works by increasing levels of serotonin (to boost mood and control appetite) and norepinephrine (to increase thermogenesis and calorie expenditure). These are effects that can also be accomplished by the use of natural products—and without the drug side effects. For example, the enhanced thermogenesis that comes from green-tea extract (discussed in Chapter 4) is primarily due to an increase of norepinephrine at the cellular level. Green-tea extracts have been shown to increase cellular norepinephrine levels and to result in an elevated metabolic rate, and at least six clinical studies have shown an enhancement of fat metabolism, overall caloric expenditure, and a promotion of weight loss following green-tea supplementation.

For the mood-balancing benefits of serotonin, a popular herbal selection is St. John's wort (900 mg/day), but because of the wide range of potential interactions between St. John's wort and virtually any prescription or over-the-counter medication, there are other, more appropriate options. One such option is an amino acid known as 5-HTP (5-hydroxytryptophan), which is the immediate precursor of serotonin. Taking 5-HTP as a daily dietary supplement can increase natural serotonin production in the brain. At least four clinical studies have shown that 5-HTP supplementation can improve mood, reduce appetite, and promote weight loss in overweight humans. See the table on page 80 for information on supplements that provide added metabolic support by increasing levels of serotonin and norepinephrine.

Chapter Highlights

◆ General metabolic support in the form of controlling thyroid hormones, serotonin, and norepinephrine can provide an added boost to other aspects of your Cortisol Connection Diet.

◆ Thyroid support must be multipronged to be effective. It must address thyroid-hormone synthesis, conversion

Dietary Supplements for Added Metabolic Support (Thyroid, Serotonin, and Norepinephrine)

Supplement	Benefits	Drawbacks	Recommended daily dosage
Guggul extract (Commiphora mukul, standardized for guggulsterones)	Thyroid support (increases T3 levels)	None	200–500 mg
Rhodiola (Rhodiola rosea, standardized for rosavins)	Thyroid support (reduces cortisol blockade of T4➠T3 conversion)	None	250–1,000 mg
Bladderwrack (Fucus vesiculosus)	Thyroid support (iodine source for T4 production)	None	100–400 mg
Selenium	Thyroid support (cofactor for 5'-deiodinase enzyme)	None	50–150 mcg
Zinc	Thyroid support (cofactor for 5'-deiodinase enzyme)	None	15–45 mg
Vitamin E (as natural d-alpha tocopherol)	Thyroid support (stabilized cell membranes, location of 5'-deiodinase enzyme)	None	30–100 IU
5-hydroxytryptophan (Griffonia simplicifolia, standardized for 5-HTP)	Serotonin support (increases serotonin levels for appetite and mood control)	None	100–400 mg
Green-tea extract (Camellia sinensis, standardized for catechins)	Norepinephrine support Increases norepinephrine levels for enhanced thermogenesis and calorie expenditure)	None	200–750 mg

of T4 to T3, and balancing of the normal stress response.

◆ Serotonin modulation can influence mood and appetite simultaneously and thus result in weight loss over time.

◆ Norepinephrine levels are a primary driver of cellular energy levels and can be increased to boost overall thermogenesis.

Mitch

Dr. Talbott's Cortisol Connection Diet has helped me to lose more than fifty-five pounds of body weight and at least six inches off my waist. Having recently lost my job due to a downsizing at work, I found that the stress and weight gain were killing me. During my job search I was frustrated every time I went for an interview because my suits were fitting tighter and tighter—especially around the waist.

Before I started on Dr. Talbott's program, my stress level was through the roof, I had just bought a bigger belt, and I was starting to eye the 46-inch-waist pants (up from my then size 44 and my usual 38). At the urging of my wife, I started on Dr. Talbott's program, figuring that I'd get a "salad and salmon diet" and be told to exercise more—but I was wrong. The program was more of a lifestyle plan than an actual diet. In fact, Dr. Talbott was encouraging most of us to eat more rather than less, in order to get our metabolic engines fired up and help us lose weight.

I can't say enough about how beneficial the program was for me. In addition to losing weight and inches, I feel a whole lot better. My mood is up and my stress is way down from where it was at the start of the program. Best of all, I have a new problem to deal with. In my new job, whenever I put on a suit for a client meeting, I have to cinch the belt extra tight because now my suits are too loose in the waist rather than too tight, as they were just a few months ago. I owe a great big thanks to Dr. Talbott for putting together a program that even a stressed-out guy who doesn't go for diet and exercise very much can follow and get results.

. . . .
.
.

CHAPTER 6

Putting It All Together

At this point, you can see the value in using diet and supplements to simultaneously affect cortisol, blood sugar, thermogenesis, thyroid function, serotonin, and norepinephrine as important metabolic control points in the regulation of body weight. This chapter presents in a convenient, usable format a plan that will help you pull all the book's suggestions together to formulate your personalized Cortisol Connection program. By following the guidelines offered here, which are based on the information presented in earlier chapters, you can customize the Cortisol Connection Diet for your needs. Doing so will provide you with the most effective approach to shedding those "last twenty pounds" of weight that are so problematic for millions of Americans.

Perhaps the most important aspect of any effective lifestyle regimen is not so much that it works, but that it works *for you*. In this way, the Cortisol Connection Diet is infinitely customizable to your own specific likes, dislikes, and preferences—which means you can use it to help guide you in crafting your own *personalized* approach to effective, long-lasting, and tasty weight loss.

Be sure to refer to the daily logs at the back of the book—and be sure to carry the logs with you for the first few weeks—to help you choose foods and meals with a high balance factor (quality) and in the right portion sizes (quantity), using the helping hand as a guide. The log can also help to remind you *when* and *what* to eat and how to supplement your diet.

In short, the practical nature of the Cortisol Connection Diet will take much of the mystery and confusion out of achieving long-lasting weight loss, because it addresses the key metabolic factors (cortisol, blood sugar, thermogenesis, serotonin, thyroid hormones, and norepinephrine) that cause most of us to gain weight and struggle with weight loss.

WHERE DOES EXERCISE FIT IN?

You may have noticed that very little has been said up to now about the role of exercise as part of the Cortisol Connection Diet. That's because the key benefit of exercise for weight control is *not* that it burns a significant number of calories. Exercise certainly burns some calories, but far fewer than you may think. Instead, the primary value of exercise as part of a weight-control regimen lies in its profound effects on improving insulin function and modulating levels of blood sugar, cortisol, and serotonin (with cortisol and serotonin control being responsible for many of the "feel-good" effects of a good workout).

The metabolic benefits of exercise are far-reaching, but from a weight-control perspective, a regular exercise program "teaches" our muscles to transport glucose more efficiently and to respond to cortisol more effectively. Exercise also improves our body's sensitivity to both insulin and cortisol, so we are able to get by with much lower levels of both of these powerful metabolic hormones and therefore avoid many of the health problems (such as weight gain) that are associated with chronically elevated levels.

An interesting side effect of optimizing your control of blood-sugar and cortisol levels is an increase both in general calorie expenditure and in fat burning (otherwise known as thermogenesis). This means that exercise *on its own* will influence, to a certain degree, each of the primary metabolic control points (MCPs) related to body-weight regulation—so get out there and do it.

Regular exercise is often promoted as a tool for preventing weight gain, and there is good evidence that people who are more active have a reduced risk of gaining weight. One study from the School of Public Health at Harvard University followed a large group of men over two years. At the beginning of the study, the most active men and those who watched fewer hours of television were less likely to be overweight, and after two years, those who were most active and who watched fewer hours of television had gained less weight. Data from several national surveys (in both the United States and other countries) clearly show that people who maintain higher levels of physical activity are less likely to gain weight or at least tend to gain less weight than their inactive counterparts.

Overall, then, whether exercise is a good tool for promoting weight *loss* is controversial. A recent scientific review of studies related to the effect of physical activity on weight loss concluded that adding exercise to a reduced-calorie diet only leads to modest additional weight loss (five to seven pounds), but that regular exercise is strongly associated with *maintenance* of weight loss. Therefore, although exercise may be a less important tool for initial weight loss, it is an important factor in the prevention of weight regain.

So, with most of the available evidence suggesting that physical activity plays a more important role in reducing age-related weight gain than it does in actually promoting weight loss, the obvious question is "Why isn't exercise more effective in promoting weight loss?" The answer is because it is simply very difficult to promote a substantial negative energy balance with exercise. Negative energy balance is the state where a person expends more energy (calories) than he or she consumes. To achieve a state of negative energy balance, one must consume fewer calories, expend more energy, or both. This seems like a pretty simple task, but the reality is that most adult Americans lack a good understanding of the energy value of different foods and exercises. Most people, including professional dieticians and physiologists, tend to underestimate the caloric value of food and overestimate the caloric value of exercise. Consider some of the values in the table below:

The energy cost of exercise versus diet

Energy (calories)	Exercise for 30 minutes*	Dietary equivalent
100	Walking, leisurely pace	3/4 cup of ice cream
150	Walking, brisk pace	6 Oreo cookies
200	Stationary cycling, easy	3 tbsp. peanut butter
240	Lap swimming, leisurely	20 potato chips
240	Aerobic exercise class	1 slice pizza
300	Lap swimming, vigorous	12 Hershey Kisses
300	Stationary cycling, vigorous	1 fried chicken leg
300	Running, slow pace	1 Burger King cheese burger
500	Running, fast pace	1 Taco Bell bean burrito with cheese

* This estimate is based on a person who weighs 175 pounds. For a person who weighs more than 175 pounds, the estimated energy expenditure is slightly higher, and it's slightly lower for someone who weighs less than 175 pounds.

As you can see, it is easy to wipe out the calories burned off by exercise with a few bites of the wrong foods. With a caloric deficit of 3,500 calories needed to lose one pound of fat, and a general goal of losing one to two pounds of fat per week (a reasonable goal for most overweight individuals), this would require a caloric deficit of 500–1,000 calories each day. For most people, this would mean thirty to sixty minutes of intense exercise daily (which I'd love to see more people doing)—but since most American adults are extremely sedentary and since about 40 percent get no physical activity, this level of exercise would be difficult to adhere to for most people.

In one study from the University of Pennsylvania, women who had lost weight were followed over the subsequent twelve months. The threshold level of exercise needed to prevent weight regain corresponded to approximately eighty minutes of brisk walking per day. People enrolled in the National Weight Control Registry (NWCR) report a similar level of activity. (The NWCR is a large database of individuals who have maintained a minimum thirty-pound weight loss for at least one year.) In addition, recent data from Japan suggest that accumulating twelve thousand to sixteen thousand steps per day (measured with pedometers) can also help to prevent weight regain.

WHAT TYPE OF EXERCISE SHOULD YOU DO?

Anything—as long as you do it! You simply need to get out there and move your body for at least three to six hours each week (30 to 60 minutes per day, six days a week). If our goal were simply to burn as many calories as possible with exercise, then we'd be shooting for as much intensity as we could stand (exercising as hard as possible for as many minutes as we could). But because our reasons for exercising go beyond a pure focus on calorie expenditure and instead focus on optimizing the six metabolic control points (cortisol, blood sugar,

thermogenesis, serotonin, thyroid hormones, and norepinephrine), our exercise efforts will focus less on intensity
(how hard you go—which is important for cardiovascular
effects) or duration (how long you go—which is important
for muscular endurance), and more on frequency (how often
you exercise, no matter your intensity or duration). In this
context (focusing on frequency), I would much rather see my
clients walking for 30 minutes, six days a week (180 minutes
for the week) than jogging for 60 minutes, three days a week
(even though that still adds up to 180 minutes for the week).

An effective approach to increasing your frequency of
exercise is to try building exercise into your daily routine.
This might mean parking a few blocks away from your work-
place and walking that last bit, doing your own yard work
instead of hiring someone else to do it, climbing the stairs to
your fourth-floor office, or rediscovering the pleasures of rid-
ing your bike for nearby errands and social visits.

If you're "too busy" to exercise (the most common
excuse for not exercising), then you need to accept the fact
that you will never lose those last twenty pounds, because
without exercise your metabolic control of blood sugar and
cortisol will never be optimized. Think about all the things in
which you invest 30 to 60 minutes each day—television,
newspapers, Internet surfing, etc.—and then ask yourself if
investing that same amount of time in your health, in your
body, and in yourself is worth it. I think we both know what
the answer will be.

SUPPLEMENTS FOR OPTIMIZING METABOLIC CONTROL AND WEIGHT LOSS

Cortisol Controllers

Select one or more of the following. Divide the dosage between morning and evening. These are especially important during periods of heightened stress.

- ◆ magnolia bark (totaling 200–800 mg/day)

- ◆ theanine (totaling 25–250 mg/day)

- ◆ beta-sitosterol (totaling 30–300 mg/day)

- ◆ phosphatidylserine (totaling 50–100 mg/day)

Blood-Sugar Controllers

Select one or more of the following. Divide the dosage among three meals.

- ◆ chromium (totaling 100–400 mcg/day)

- ◆ vanadium (totaling 10–100 mcg/day)

- ◆ banaba leaf (totaling 10–100 mg/day)

Thermogenesis Boosters

Take one or both of the following. Divide the dosage between morning and midday.

- ◆ green-tea extract (totaling 200–750 mg/day)

- ◆ calcium (500–750 mg as a supplement, for a total of 1,200–1,500 mg/day)

General Metabolic Support

Select one or more for thyroid support, plus one each for serotonin and norepinephrine support. Take with the midday meal.

- ◆ guggul extract (totaling 200–500 mg/day for thyroid support)

- ◆ rhodiola (totaling 250–1,000 mg/day for cortisol/stress control and energy)

- ◆ bladderwrack (totaling 100–400 mg/day for thyroid support)

- ◆ selenium (totaling 50–150 mcg/day for thyroid support)

- ◆ zinc (totaling 15–45 mg/day for thyroid support)

- ◆ vitamin E (totaling 30–100 IU/day for thyroid support, but see below for recommended dosage as an antioxidant)

- ◆ 5-HTP (totaling 100–400 mg/day for serotonin support)

- ◆ green-tea extract (totaling 200–750 mg/day for norepinephrine support)

Multivitamin/Mineral and Antioxidant Supplements

Take these every day with meals, especially when following a thermogenic regimen.

- ◆ calcium (500–750 mg as a supplement, for a total of 1,200–1,500 mg/day for cortisol control and thermogenesis)

- ◆ magnesium (125–250 mg/day for cortisol control)

- B-complex vitamins (2–10 mg/day *of each* for cortisol control)

- chromium (50–200 mcg/day for blood-sugar control)

- vanadium (10–30 mcg/day for blood-sugar control)

- vitamin C (100–500 mg/day for cortisol control and antioxidant effects)

- vitamin E (200–400 IU/day for antioxidant effects)

- thiols (10–100 mg/day *total* of antioxidants, such as selenium, cysteine, alpha-lipoic acid)

- carotenoids (10–30 mg/day *total* of antioxidants, such as beta-carotene, lycopene, lutein)

- flavonoids (100–300 mg/day total of antioxidants, such as catechins, polyphenols, quercetin, isoflavones)

SAMPLE MENU PLAN FOR MEALS AND SNACKS

Remember from Chapter 1 that we need to space out our meals and snacks throughout the day to help regulate blood-sugar and cortisol metabolism. Follow the general plan outlined in the table on pages 92–93 and the "Further Guidelines" below, but substitute foods that you prefer (e.g., turkey for roast beef on your sandwich or sushi instead of salmon at dinner) or foods that you have ready access to (such as when eating away from home).

Further Guidelines

Number of portions: A *snack* consists of **one** appropriately sized serving from the fruit/veggie group, plus **one** appropri-

Sample Menu Plan

Time	Meal	Fruit/ Veggie	Starch	Protein	Fat	Supplements
7 A.M.	Snack	Banana	N/A	N/A	Peanut butter	☑ 8 oz. water
9 A.M.	Breakfast	Grapefruit (+2 teaspoons of added sugar, optional)	Shredded wheat cereal	1% milk	Coffee with half & half	☑ Multivitamin ☑ Cortisol ☑ Blood sugar ☑ Thermo ☑ 8 oz. water
Noon	Snack	Apple	N/A	N/A	Block of cheese	☑ 8 oz. water
2 P.M.	Lunch	3 tomato slices 1 leaf Romaine lettuce; 1 pear	2 slices whole-wheat bread	Lean roast beef	Swiss cheese and mustard to taste	☑ Blood sugar ☑ Thermo ☑ 8 oz. water

Sample Menu Plan (cont'd.)

Time	Meal	Fruit/ Veggie	Starch	Protein	Fat	Supplements
5 P.M.	Snack	Baby carrots	N/A	N/A	Salad dressing	☑ 8 oz. water
7 P.M.	Dinner	½ cup of green beans; ½ cup of carrots	1 whole-wheat dinner roll	Salmon fillet seasoned with olive oil and garlic	Olive oil with garlic (for the roll and fish)	☑ Multivitamin ☑ Cortisol ☑ Blood sugar
9 P.M.	Dessert*	Air-popped popcorn	N/A	N/A	Melted butter	☑ 8 oz. water

* (see "Further Guidelines" on page 94)

Did you exercise today? What did you do? How did you feel?

_____

_____

_____

Total minutes of exercise _____   How much sleep did you get last night? _____

ately sized serving of fat. A *meal* consists of **one** appropriately sized serving from **each** of the starch, protein, and fat groups, plus **one or two** appropriately sized servings from the fruit/veggie group.

Fluids: An 8-ounce glass of water is suggested with each meal and snack. (8 fluid ounces = 1 cup.)

Sleep prescription: 10:30 P.M. to 6:00 A.M.—i.e., get at least 7.5 hours nightly for optimal cortisol control.

Exercise prescription: 30–60 minutes of activity, six times per week, for optimal insulin sensitivity and blood-sugar control.

Fruit/veggie guideline: Remember, "Choose it if it's bright, and forget it if it's white." This will guide you toward brightly colored choices that are better sources of antioxidants and essential phytonutrients.

Starch guideline: Select dark, thick, course, chewy, and minimally processed forms of grains over their highly refined counterparts (white, light, smooth, puffed, and fluffy).

Protein guideline: Choose lean cuts of meat, poultry, pork, and fish.

Fat guideline: Don't skip fat to save a few calories; instead, add it to meals and snacks as a metabolic regulator. Avoid trans-fats in the form of hydrogenated oils in processed foods.

Dessert guideline (bonus!): If you have exercised for 30–60 minutes on a particular day, then as an optional fourth snack of the day add either a cocktail or a glass of wine or beer with dinner, or a fist-sized dessert. If you have not exercised, then skip the alcohol and end dinner with a piece of fresh fruit instead.

Following the Cortisol Connection Diet helps you balance the *quality* of your food choices (the balance factor) with the *quantity* of those choices (the helping-hand guidelines), so you regulate calories to approximately 1,500 per day from a balanced intake of about 55 percent carbohydrates, 20 percent protein, and 25 percent fat. Remember that these are exactly the levels associated with the most dramatic weight loss and longest-lasting weight maintenance.

In Closing

That brings us to the end of *The Cortisol Connection Diet*. I hope that at this point you feel as strongly as I do that the Cortisol Connection approach to weight loss is the most practical and easy-to-follow approach to using food to control the effects of cortisol and glucose in your body—and ultimately to controlling how many calories you burn off or store as fat. It is my sincere wish that you use this book and its many recommendations to help you make the Cortisol Connection a part of your everyday life.

Remember to use the sample menus and supplement suggestions located in this chapter, and the list of frequently asked questions (FAQ) located in Appendix B. The daily logs at the back of the book should be your daily diet companion for at least the first few weeks of your journey into the Cortisol Connection approach to metabolic control. Carry it with you to help you choose foods and meals with a high balance factor and an appropriate serving size (helping hand), and to remind you when to eat and how to supplement your diet.

Following the Cortisol Connection Diet will help to control your appetite, promote fat loss, and simply make you feel great—with more energy, better mental focus, a better body, and a better you. Thanks for reading.

. . . .
:
.

Putting the Cortisol Connection Diet to the Test

As a scientist I find that theories and ideas are nice, but cold hard evidence is where the rubber meets the road. In the words of many of my colleagues, I want to "see the data" about a particular program before I will believe it works. Based on the data, other professionals can recommend a given program with a certain degree of confidence that it will actually work for their clients and patients. So before releasing this book, I felt very strongly that I had to put the Cortisol Connection Diet to the test to see if these ideas would really stand up to the harsh reality of losing weight in the real world. It all makes sense on paper from a biochemical and physiological perspective, but there have been lots of great ideas on paper that never made a lick of difference to anyone in the real world.

With the general plan for the Cortisol Connection Diet developed, and with the invaluable assistance of AnneMarie Christopulos at the Treehouse Athletic Club in Draper, Utah, fifty motivated volunteers set out with me on a twelve-week journey to see if this program was all it seemed. The program lasted for twelve weeks because we wanted to see how people felt after following it for several months. Almost any program, no matter how tedious and restrictive, can be followed for a few weeks, but sticking with something for a full three months means that it has a high likelihood of becoming a lifestyle rather than simply a temporary diet.

One important aspect of the program was that we set out to recruit as many hard cases as we could find. By "hard cases" I mean people who in the past had tried and tried and tried to lose weight with other programs and who just could not seem to succeed. Why would we recruit the toughest cases and set ourselves up for failure? Simply because in my experience conducting weight-loss trials over the past decade or so, it is easy to recruit a group of overweight subjects and get them to lose large amounts of weight in a short period of time—and almost any simplified program of diet or exercise will do it. With the Cortisol Connection Diet, I'm trying to help the millions of Americans who struggle day in and day out with that ten or twenty or thirty pounds of weight that simply won't respond to simplified diets and exercise regimens. It's these folks who need help cracking their weight-loss code—and the Cortisol Connection Diet was put to the test to help them.

Over the twelve weeks, we met as a group on six occasions—approximately every other week—to talk about one of the six metabolic control points: cortisol, blood sugar, thermogenesis, serotonin, thyroid hormones, and norepinephrine. We also talked about how diet, exercise, and supplements could have an impact. Over the three months, we measured body weight, body fat, waist circumference, cortisol levels, and stress/anxiety levels. Using a double-blind, placebo-controlled study design, we also studied whether or not people taking a dietary supplement for cortisol and blood-sugar control in addition to their diet and exercise program might lose more weight (or have an easier time of it) compared to a group taking a placebo or nothing at all.

The results were nothing short of dramatic. Not only did virtually every person in the program lose body weight, body fat, and inches around their midsection, but the majority of people also reported increased feelings of energy, reduced stress/anxiety, control of appetite and cravings, and no feelings of deprivation. The most common comment was that nobody felt like they were on a "diet," and yet they continued to lose weight, fat, and inches. Plus, they felt great doing it.

Of particular interest over the twelve weeks was the fact that members of the group taking the dietary supplement for cortisol and blood-sugar control (in addition to following the diet and exercise prescriptions) lost about 20 percent more weight/fat and almost double the inches from their waists than did members of the group following diet and exercise alone. In no way does this mean that the supplement was a substitute for diet and exercise, but it suggests strongly that by adding the supplement to their diet and exercise regimen, they were able to reap some additional metabolic control and thus enjoy a greater degree of weight loss. In many ways, the results make perfect sense, because the people in the supplement group had three factors driving them toward weight loss (diet, exercise, supplements), while the placebo group had only two (diet and exercise). No matter what group each subject was in, however, the more attention he or she paid to controlling those six metabolic control points, the more of those stubborn "last twenty pounds" they were able to lose, even after having struggled with those pounds for so long.

The fact that a new "popular" diet (that is, one written for the real world and for real people) was being studied ahead of its publication was quite a surprise to most of my colleagues. The typical chain of events is for some diet guru to write a book with lots of miraculous claims (eat all you want and lose weight!), for the author and publisher to hook up with a marketing outfit, and for the book to ride the best-seller charts until people figure out that it doesn't really work as promised after all. In the case of the Cortisol Connection Diet, I was prepared to put my money where my mouth was so that when my colleagues said, "Show me the data," I could do just that. The data from our fifty-subject, twelve-week program was accepted for presentation and publication at the Fifth International Congress on Nutrition and Fitness in 2004 in Athens, Greece, perhaps one of the most prestigious scientific meetings concerning metabolism and the very metabolic control points addressed by the Cortisol Connection Diet.

Attendees at the meeting—people who came from around the world—found that the most interesting feature of the Cortisol Connection Diet was not any single aspect of the program, but rather that the synergy between the component parts was so effective when melded into a single approach. For example, we've known for years that regular exercise and a balanced diet are the foundation of a healthy weight-management program, but what the Cortisol Connection Diet showed was that by building on that diet/exercise foundation with attention to the MCPs (cortisol, blood sugar, thermogenesis, serotonin, thyroid hormones, and norepinephrine), the "standard" weight-loss results of diet plus exercise could be optimized, much to the delight of Cortisol Connection adherents.

Toward the end of the twelve-week program, some of the participants started talking about how the combination of diet, exercise, and MCPs in the Cortisol Connection Diet had put them into what they called the "sweet spot"—where their weight loss became effortless. In tennis, the sweet spot is the part of the racquet that generates the greatest velocity with the least effort; that is, you hit the ball with the same force, but it *takes off*. In rowing, we call the same phenomenon "swing"; it's where everything comes together and the boat just *cruises* along, almost with effortless grace. For a diet program to be generating the same feelings in participants was certainly something exciting. While we knew from the outset that the diet made biochemical sense "on paper," we now know that the Cortisol Connection Diet also makes sense in the real world.

. . . .
.
.

Frequently Asked Questions (FAQ)

EXERCISE

Q What are effective forms of exercise?

A All types of exercise are beneficial for overall health, but different types of exercise will deliver a different set of specific benefits. For example, aerobic exercises such as walking, jogging, cycling, and swimming tend to provide health benefits for the cardiovascular and respiratory systems, and also improve muscular endurance. Strength training, also known as resistance training, tends to provide benefits for muscular strength, bone health, and related areas. Both types of exercise are beneficial for weight loss (via an improvement in insulin sensitivity).

Q What kind of fitness program is best for a beginner?

A For beginning exercisers, and for most people who exercise for general health reasons (including weight loss), the "best" fitness program is determined by two major factors. The first is that it should combine a *variety* of exercises, including aerobic and strength activities (to provide a range of health benefits to the heart, lungs, muscles, and bones).

The second factor is that the activities need to be *enjoyable* enough for you to do them on a regular basis (several times each week).

Q **What are the most important things to remember when beginning an exercise program?**

A Start slowly, progressively build your intensity and duration, and pay attention to your body for signs that you are adequately recovering and continuing to adapt to your program.

Q **What are important things to remember in maintaining an exercise program?**

A Stick with it, because the most dramatic results come with time. Also, be prepared at some point in your fitness program to experience a plateau in the results that you're achieving—and when this happens, be ready to alter your regimen slightly. For example, one of the most effective approaches to avoiding these plateaus is to keep your body "guessing" by changing your fitness program around on a regular basis (about every six weeks).

Q **Are different forms of exercise better for some people than they are for others?**

A That depends on your fitness goals. If your primary fitness goal is to build muscle, then strength-training exercises will be your most important focus. Individuals who are trying to enhance cardiovascular fitness, however, will benefit more from aerobic exercises. If you are trying to lose body fat, then a combination of strength training and aerobic exercise will provide the best overall effect.

NUTRITION

Q **What are the side effects associated with the Atkins Diet (low carb/high protein)?**

A It depends on how the diet is approached. For example, an "Atkins" meal composed of salmon and green salad has no side effects (and obviously has many health benefits)—but an "Atkins" meal composed of a bacon double cheeseburger (hold the bun) is not good for your heart or for your waistline. Eating too much protein, which can be a problem with some versions of low-carb diets, can lead to dehydration (water loss that is often confused with weight/fat loss)—and dehydration can slow the metabolic rate and make weight maintenance more difficult. Too much protein in the diet can also displace other important food sources: If you've filled up on meat and cheese, you may not have room left to eat your salad, so the diet may fail to provide enough of many vitamins, minerals, and phytonutrients, and may also be lacking in fiber.

Q **What are the side effects associated with the ephedra diet (herbal stimulants)?**

A Diet plans based on ephedra (ma huang) and related herbal stimulants, such as caffeine (guarana, kola nut), can certainly suppress appetite and result in short-term weight loss via reduced food intake. The problems with using these herbal stimulants as weight-loss agents are many, including heart palpitations, insomnia, and elevated blood pressure, among others. In addition, herbal stimulants are known to increase cortisol levels, so the long-term effects of ephedra-type regimens are to actually *increase* appetite and body fat (via cortisol elevation).

Q What are the side effects associated with meal-replacement diets (liquid diets)?

A When used appropriately to control portion sizes and caloric intake, meal replacements are one of the easiest, safest, and most effective approaches to weight loss. Unfortunately, some meal-replacement regimens are inappropriate for long-term use, such as those that provide insufficient calories for prolonged use or those that may fail to deliver sufficient levels of important vitamins and minerals. Also, a prolonged adherence to a restrictive regimen of meal replacements (e.g., three liquid meals per day) is difficult to follow for a prolonged period of time.

SUPPLEMENTS

Q What effects do typical appetite suppressants have on the heart, and why are they dangerous?

A Typical appetite suppressants, such as ephedra and caffeine, can affect the heart in a number of adverse ways, two of which are by increasing blood pressure and heart rate. The danger with these types of side effects is that people with any risk factor for cardiovascular disease are put at additional risk.

Q How does the thermogenic effect of green tea work? Can it keep you awake at night if you take it in the evening?

A The thermogenic effect of green-tea extract has been measured as an increase in basal metabolic rate—otherwise known as the body's basic caloric expenditure. The exact mechanism for this calorie-burning effect is unknown, but several clinical studies have shown a significant increase in metabolic rate that is clearly *not* due to a stimulation of the central nervous system. This means that although metabolic rate is increased when a person regularly supplements with green-tea extract, there is no risk of stimulant-related side effects such as insomnia, heart palpitations, and elevated blood pressure.

Q Do I *have* to add a daily multivitamin to the other targeted supplements in the Cortisol Connection Diet?

A Adding a well-balanced multivitamin/mineral supplement will enhance the overall effects of the Cortisol Connection Diet through a variety of mechanisms. For example, a balanced multi will provide additional vitamins and minerals involved in optimal blood-sugar control (chromium, vanadium, alpha-lipoic acid, etc.). It will also provide important nutrients for optimal cortisol control (calcium, magnesium, vitamin C, and B-complex vitamins). In addition, although they are not related to weight-loss issues, antioxidants are important for overall health and wellness (especially when thermogenesis is increased). As such, your multi should also provide an optimal "antioxidant network" formulation, with effective levels of ingredients in each major antioxidant category (vitamins C and E, thiols, flavonoids, and carotenoids).

Q If a person wants to accelerate the system, is there anything they can do in terms of additional supplementation?

A No—this is as good as it gets with a natural approach to metabolic control. An additional way to "accelerate" the overall weight-loss effects of the Cortisol Connection Diet would be to adhere to a regimen of balanced and scientifically validated meal replacements. There are several examples of products that have been shown (without any changes in diet/exercise) to help control appetite, modulate blood-sugar levels, reduce cholesterol and triglyceride levels, and reduce body fat by two to four pounds per week. When looking for a meal replacement product (MRP), you'll want to select one that is "balanced" in its macronutrient profile (one that provides carbs, protein, fat, and fiber).

Stay away from products that provide a lot of carbohydrates without balancing those carbs with protein, and also steer clear of the high-protein products that skimp on carbs. In a 200- to 250-calorie MRP bar or shake, you'll be looking for about 20–30 grams of carbohydrate (80–120 calories), 20–40 grams of protein (80–120 calories), and 2–10 grams each of fat (18–90 calories) and fiber (no calories). Finally, check the ingredient listing of the MRP and avoid any products that contain high fructose corn syrup or hydrogenated oils (both of which will interfere with cortisol and insulin metabolism and make weight loss more difficult).

Q **Would it be harmful to double the dosages of recommended supplements? Would doing so accelerate the weight-loss effects of the Cortisol Connection Diet?**

A It is unnecessary to increase the recommended amounts of supplements. Adding more will not improve or accelerate the plan's weight-loss effects or metabolic control. With any natural product, it is important to take the products as directed—so one of the most important aspects of the Cortisol Connection Diet will be for people to take their supplements as recommended and not to randomly start popping pills at different doses and in different combinations. Refer to Chapter 6 for a sample regimen for breakfast, lunch, dinner, snacks, and supplements.

GENERAL

Q **How does the Cortisol Connection Diet affect the body's metabolism?**

A The Cortisol Connection Diet helps to modulate six of the most important metabolic factors related to weight maintenance: thermogenesis (by boosting calorie expenditure), blood sugar (by controlling appetite and carb cravings), cortisol (by alleviating the detrimental effects of elevated cortisol levels, which include increased appetite, enhanced fat storage, and disrupted blood-sugar control), serotonin (by modulating mood and appetite), thyroid hormones (by stimulating overall metabolic rate), and norepinephrine (by enhancing cellular energy levels).

Q Is the effect the same if I don't follow one of the steps (say, cortisol control)? In other words, if I just want to stimulate my metabolism, is it enough to just take the green-tea extract, or should I follow the other steps as well? Is there really a synergistic effect?

A The combined effect of each piece of the Cortisol Connection Diet will be optimized when they are all followed simultaneously. There are certainly beneficial effects delivered by each individual part of the program, but the optimal approach for weight loss is to simultaneously target multiple aspects of metabolism to deliver a true synergistic effect.

As such, cortisol control is the first step because it removes the "cortisol blockade" of optimal insulin function—which leads to better blood-sugar control (more fat burning), appetite modulation (control of carbohydrate cravings), and mobilization of fat stores.

Even with better control of insulin function and blood-sugar metabolism (through cortisol control), many people will still need additional blood-sugar control at mealtimes. This is where sugar modulation comes in—to help keep blood-sugar levels within normal ranges in the minutes to hours following meals. By keeping blood sugar within normal ranges, scientific research tells us that hunger is better managed and fat loss is optimized.

Finally, even with optimal cortisol control and optimal blood-sugar control, many people will also benefit from an increase in thermogenesis and a balancing of serotonin, thyroid hormones, and norepinephrine, so additional calories will be expended throughout the day and weight-loss efforts will be enhanced.

Q After I lose what I need to lose, what is the maintenance program? Do I need to continue the system, or is there a modified program?

A Continue with the program, but modify it according to your specific needs. For example, upon reaching your ideal body weight or your target weight, you can continue using the balance-factor and helping-hand approaches to eating in a modified fashion. For some people, this may mean a continued regimen directed toward managing stress and cortisol levels. For others, the focus may be to control blood-sugar levels within a normal range and manage carbohydrate cravings following mealtimes. These modifications will very much depend on the specific needs of the individual.

Q So how do I determine what my specific needs are?

A Ask yourself a few simple questions about your current lifestyle as it relates to control of cortisol, blood sugar, and the other MCPs. For example, if you are experiencing a heightened level of emotional stress, any lack of sleep, or any concern about your diet, then you may want to focus on cortisol control. If you find yourself craving carbohydrates or getting sleepy in the afternoon, then you may want to focus on blood-sugar control. If you find that you tend to feel cold during the day (a low body temperature) or feel mentally or physically sluggish, then you may want to focus on boosting thermogenesis and balancing your thyroid hormones and norepinephrine. If you feel that your mood is lower than it should be, then you may consider focusing on balancing your serotonin.

Q How about the person who exercises regularly and eats right, but still can't seem to lose those "last twenty pounds" he or she has been carrying for years? Will this help?

A This person is the perfect candidate for the Cortisol Connection Diet! The last twenty pounds tend to be the hardest to lose because they result from simultaneous metabolic changes in the areas of blood-sugar and cortisol metabolism. Only by simultaneously optimizing those aspects of metabolism can people realistically hope to achieve their ultimate weight-loss goals. For example, a person could be following the "perfect" diet and exercise regimen, but because of metabolic dysregulation of blood sugar, insulin, and cortisol, they are unable to lose those last few pounds. Upon optimizing these metabolic parameters, their "perfect" diet and exercise regimen can now have its desired effects.

Q Does the Cortisol Connection Diet offer a benefit for people with syndrome X?

A Absolutely. Numerous scientific publications show that cortisol overexposure is directly related to syndrome X and that most aspects of the Cortisol Connection Diet are effective in controlling many of the metabolic features and reducing the progression of the side effects associated with syndrome X.

Q What can I expect to see, feel, and notice after I have been following the Cortisol Connection Diet for a few weeks?

A
- less tension
- better mental focus
- more restful sleep
- fewer/reduced cravings
- no hunger
- enhanced stamina
- general feelings of well-being
- weight loss

Q What kind of timetable can I expect for results?

A Results will vary from one individual to another. Some people will lose substantial amounts of weight and body fat in a short period of time, while others will require several weeks or months to notice substantial benefits. In most cases, however, normal, healthy people who have been following the Cortisol Connection Diet have reported noticeable benefits in the areas of tension, appetite, and weight control within a few days.

Resources

The Cortisol Connection: Why Stress Makes You Fat and Ruins Your Health—and What You Can Do about It, by Shawn M. Talbott, Ph.D. (Alameda, CA: Hunter House, 2002).

A *Guide to Understanding Dietary Supplements*, by Shawn M. Talbott, Ph.D. (Binghamton, NY: Haworth Press, 2003).

Eat, Drink, and Be Healthy, by Walter C. Willett, M.D. (New York, NY: Fireside/Simon and Schuster, 2001).

Eating for Optimum Health, by Andrew Weil, M.D. (New York, NY: Random House, 2000).

SupplementWatch website: www.supplementwatch.com. Offers unbiased educational information about dietary supplement use (or avoidance). (Note: Shawn M. Talbott was one of the founders of Supplement Watch and has contributed extensively to the website.)

Daily Logs

The daily log pages that follow will enable you to track your progress with the Cortisol Connection Diet. One week of log pages is provided here, and you can download additional blank log pages from the Hunter House website (www.hunterhouse.com) or at the Cortisol Connection Diet website (www.cortisoldiet.com).

On each log page, you will track your daily food and supplement intake as well as your duration of exercise and sleep. Your log pages start on Monday and end on Sunday. You should note your body weight on Monday, but not on other days of the week (instead of weighing yourself every day, try to focus on how tight or loose your clothes are fitting—especially around the waist where you will be losing the greatest amount of body fat). Be sure to take your weight early in the morning.

Be sure to refer to the Sample Menu Plan on pages 92–93 to get an idea of how to fill out your pages.

Your log pages will be most useful to you if you actually carry them with you for the first week. This will remind you to choose "high-balance-factor" meals, to take your supplements, and to adhere to your exercise regimen. By "logging" your diet and exercise patterns for a single week you'll become more familiar with the balance-factor approach to weight loss, and it will soon become a natural part of your daily routine.

"Quit worrying about your health—and it will go away." — Robert Orben

Sample Menu Plan   Week 1 / 2 / 3 / ____   MONDAY   Body weight ____

Time	Meal	Fruit/ Veggie	Starch	Protein	Fat	Supplements
7 A.M.	Snack					☐ 8 oz. water
9 A.M.	Breakfast					☐ Multivitamin ☐ Cortisol ☐ Blood sugar ☐ Thermo ☐ 8 oz. water
Noon	Snack					☐ 8 oz. water
2 P.M.	Lunch					☐ Blood sugar ☐ Thermo ☐ 8 oz. water

Sample Menu Plan Week 1 / 2 / 3 / _____ MONDAY

Time	Meal	Fruit/ Veggie	Starch	Protein	Fat	Supplements
5 P.M.	Snack					☐ 8 oz. water
7 P.M.	Dinner					☐ Multivitamin ☐ Cortisol ☐ Blood sugar
9 P.M.	Dessert					☐ 8 oz. water

Did you exercise today? What did you do? How did you feel?

_____

_____

Total minutes of exercise _____   How much sleep did you get last night? _____

"Stick to the present and the future. Look to the past only when you can do it rationally and objectively as a way to improve on the other two." — Daniel Meachum

Sample Menu Plan **Week 1 / 2 / 3 / ____** **TUESDAY**

Time	Meal	Fruit/ Veggie	Starch	Protein	Fat	Supplements
7 A.M.	Snack					☐ 8 oz. water
9 A.M.	Breakfast					☐ Multivitamin ☐ Cortisol ☐ Blood sugar ☐ Thermo ☐ 8 oz. water
Noon	Snack					☐ 8 oz. water
2 P.M.	Lunch					☐ Blood sugar ☐ Thermo ☐ 8 oz. water

Sample Menu Plan   Week 1 / 2 / 3 / ___   TUESDAY

Time	Meal	Fruit/ Veggie	Starch	Protein	Fat	Supplements
5 P.M.	Snack					☐ 8 oz. water
7 P.M.	Dinner					☐ Multivitamin ☐ Cortisol ☐ Blood sugar
9 P.M.	Dessert					☐ 8 oz. water

Did you exercise today? What did you do? How did you feel?

_____

_____

_____

Total minutes of exercise _____   How much sleep did you get last night? _____

"If you're alive, you got to flap your arms and legs, you got to jump around a lot,
because life is the very opposite of death." — Mel Brooks

Sample Menu Plan   Week 1 / 2 / 3 / _____   WEDNESDAY

Time	Meal	Fruit/ Veggie	Starch	Protein	Fat	Supplements
7 A.M.	Snack					☐ 8 oz. water
9 A.M.	Breakfast					☐ Multivitamin ☐ Cortisol ☐ Blood sugar ☐ Thermo ☐ 8 oz. water
Noon	Snack					☐ 8 oz. water
2 P.M.	Lunch					☐ Blood sugar ☐ Thermo ☐ 8 oz. water

Sample Menu Plan   Week 1 / 2 / 3 / ____   WEDNESDAY

Time	Meal	Fruit/ Veggie	Starch	Protein	Fat	Supplements
5 P.M.	Snack					☐ 8 oz. water
7 P.M.	Dinner					☐ Multivitamin ☐ Cortisol ☐ Blood sugar
9 P.M.	Dessert					☐ 8 oz. water

Did you exercise today? What did you do? How did you feel?

_____

_____

Total minutes of exercise _____   How much sleep did you get last night? _____

"If anything is sacred, the human body is sacred." — Walt Whitman

Sample Menu Plan   Week 1 / 2 / 3 / ____   THURSDAY

Time	Meal	Fruit/ Veggie	Starch	Protein	Fat	Supplements
7 A.M.	Snack					☐ 8 oz. water
9 A.M.	Breakfast					☐ Multivitamin ☐ Cortisol ☐ Blood sugar ☐ Thermo ☐ 8 oz. water
Noon	Snack					☐ 8 oz. water
2 P.M.	Lunch					☐ Blood sugar ☐ Thermo ☐ 8 oz. water

Sample Menu Plan   Week 1 / 2 / 3 / ____   THURSDAY

Time	Meal	Fruit/Veggie	Starch	Protein	Fat	Supplements
5 P.M.	Snack					☐ 8 oz. water
7 P.M.	Dinner					☐ Multivitamin ☐ Cortisol ☐ Blood sugar
9 P.M.	Dessert					☐ 8 oz. water

Did you exercise today? What did you do? How did you feel?

_____

Total minutes of exercise _____   How much sleep did you get last night? _____

"There is no cure for birth and death—save to enjoy the interval." — George Santayana

Sample Menu Plan   Week 1 / 2 / 3 / ____   FRIDAY

Time	Meal	Fruit/Veggie	Starch	Protein	Fat	Supplements
7 A.M.	Snack					☐ 8 oz. water
9 A.M.	Breakfast					☐ Multivitamin ☐ Cortisol ☐ Blood sugar ☐ Thermo ☐ 8 oz. water
Noon	Snack					☐ 8 oz. water
2 P.M.	Lunch					☐ Blood sugar ☐ Thermo ☐ 8 oz. water

Sample Menu Plan		Week 1 / 2 / 3 / _____		FRIDAY		
Time	Meal	Fruit/ Veggie	Starch	Protein	Fat	Supplements
5 P.M.	Snack					☐ 8 oz. water
7 P.M.	Dinner					☐ Multivitamin ☐ Cortisol ☐ Blood sugar
9 P.M.	Dessert					☐ 8 oz. water

Did you exercise today? What did you do? How did you feel?

_____

_____

_____

Total minutes of exercise _____   How much sleep did you get last night? _____

"Knowing is not enough; we must apply. Willing is not enough; we must do."
— Johann Wolfgang von Goethe

Sample Menu Plan   Week 1 / 2 / 3 / _____   SATURDAY

Time	Meal	Fruit/ Veggie	Starch	Protein	Fat	Supplements
7 A.M.	Snack					☐ 8 oz. water
9 A.M.	Breakfast					☐ Multivitamin ☐ Cortisol ☐ Blood sugar ☐ Thermo ☐ 8 oz. water
Noon	Snack					☐ 8 oz. water
2 P.M.	Lunch					☐ Blood sugar ☐ Thermo ☐ 8 oz. water

Sample Menu Plan   Week 1 / 2 / 3 / ____   SATURDAY

Time	Meal	Fruit/ Veggie	Starch	Protein	Fat	Supplements
5 P.M.	Snack					☐ 8 oz. water
7 P.M.	Dinner					☐ Multivitamin ☐ Cortisol ☐ Blood sugar
9 P.M.	Dessert					☐ 8 oz. water

Did you exercise today? What did you do? How did you feel?

_____

Total minutes of exercise _____   How much sleep did you get last night? _____

"Becoming a star may not be your destiny, but being the best that you can be is a goal that you can set for yourself." — Bryan Lindsay

Sample Menu Plan   Week 1 / 2 / 3 / _____   **SUNDAY**

Time	Meal	Fruit/Veggie	Starch	Protein	Fat	Supplements
7 A.M.	Snack					☐ 8 oz. water
9 A.M.	Breakfast					☐ Multivitamin ☐ Cortisol ☐ Blood sugar ☐ Thermo ☐ 8 oz. water
Noon	Snack					☐ 8 oz. water
2 P.M.	Lunch					☐ Blood sugar ☐ Thermo ☐ 8 oz. water

Sample Menu Plan   Week 1 / 2 / 3 / ___   SUNDAY

Time	Meal	Fruit/ Veggie	Starch	Protein	Fat	Supplements
5 P.M.	Snack					☐ 8 oz. water
7 P.M.	Dinner					☐ Multivitamin ☐ Cortisol ☐ Blood sugar
9 P.M.	Dessert					☐ 8 oz. water

Did you exercise today? What did you do? How did you feel?

_____

_____

Total minutes of exercise _____   How much sleep did you get last night? _____

Index

A

additives, food
    high-fructose corn syrup, 18–20
    hydrogenated oils, 20–21
aging, and metabolic rates, 57–58
American Journal of Clinical Nutrition, 19, 67
antioxidants, 62–63
appetite suppression, 77–79, 105
Atkins Diet, 8, 9, 41, 104
Ayurvedic medicine, 77

B

balance factor, 11–12, 24–25
balance index. *See* balance factor
banaba leaf, 51, 52
beta-sitosterol, 34, 35
blood sugar, 15, 24, 39–55
    controlling with supplements, 50–52, 53
    and cortisol, 44–45
    and the glycemic index, 47–50
    and insulin, 42–44
breads, whole-grain, 12–13
breakfast, importance of, 60–61

C

caffeine, 64–65, 68
calcium, 65–67
calories
    burned through exercise, 86
    recommended, 24
    restriction of, 8, 61
carbohydrates, 94
    complex vs. simple, 49–50
    portion size, 16
    quality of, 12–13
carotenoids, 63
catechins, 68
Chinese medicine, 70, 77
cholesterol, 20
Christopulos, AnneMarie, 97
chromium, 51
cortisol, 24, 27–38
    and blood sugar, 44–45, 54
    controlling with supplements, 34–36
    metabolic effects of elevated levels, 30
    and stress, 28–29
Cortisol Connection, The (Talbott), 33

D

daily logs, 113–127
dehydration, 62
deiodination, 76
desserts, 94
diet personality, 41–42
diets, 6–7
    Atkins, 41, 104
    long-range effectiveness, 8–9
    low-carbohydrate, 8–9, 39–40
    low-fat, 9, 39–40
    meal-replacement (liquid), 105
    Ornish, 41
    and stress, 31–32
    success rates of, 40–41
    Weight Watchers, 41
    Zone, 41

E

Endocrinology, 78
ephedra (ma huang), 64–65, 104
exercise, 84–88, 94, 102–103
    frequency of, 86
    and weight loss, 85

F

fat, dietary, 94
    hydrogenated oils, 20–21
    portion control, 17
    quality of, 14–15
fiber, 15
    from whole foods, 13
5-HTP, 79
flavonoids, 63
foods
    balancing, 11–12, 24–25
    portion control, 15–17, 94
    quality analysis of, 12–15
    whole, 12–13
    See also carbohydrates; fat,
        dietary; protein
forskolin, 64–65
free radicals, 62–63, 72
fructose, 18–20

G

glycemic index (GI), 47–50, 54
glycemic load (GL), 47–50
green tea, 67–69, 79, 105
guggul, 77

H

high-fructose corn syrup (HFCS),
    18–20
hydrogenated oils, 20–21
hyperthyroidism, 75–76
hypothyroidism, 75–76

I

insulin, 19, 42–44
insulin resistance, 19, 43, 44

L

leptin, 19, 43
low-carbohydrate diet, 8–9, 39–40
low-fat diet, 9, 39–40

M

ma huang, 64–65, 104
magnolia bark, 34, 35
maintenance program (diet), 109
meal plans, 91–94
Meridia (albutramine), 78
metabolic adaptation, 2–3
metabolic control points (MCPs),
    3–4, 42
metabolic regulator, 14, 15
metabolic support, 74–82
    norepinephrine, 77–79
    serotonin, 77–79
    thyroid, 75–77
metabolic systems, 9–10, 24
multivitamin supplements, 34, 106

N

New England Journal of Medicine,
    40
non-selective sympathomimetic,
    69
norepinephrine, 10, 24, 77–79
nutrition. *See* foods

O

obesity, 19
oils, hydrogenated, 20–21
Ornish Diet, 8, 9, 41

P

Paleo Diet, 8
partially hydrogenated oils, 20–21
phosphatidylserine, 34, 35
portion control, 15–17, 94
Pritikin Diet, 8
protein, 94
    portion control, 16
    quality of, 13–14

Protein Power Diet, 8
Psychoneuroendocrinology, 78

Q

quality analysis (of food), 12–15

R

resting metabolic rate (RMR), 2
rhodiola, 77

S

satiety, 15
semi-selective sympathomimetic, 69
SENSE program, 33, 37
serotonin, 9–10, 24, 77–79
sleep, 44–45, 54, 94
snacks, 22, 94
South Beach Diet, 8, 9
St. John's wort, 79
stress, 27–32, 36, 37
   and appetite, 78
   and cortisol levels, 28–32
   and dieting, 31–32
sucrose, 18–20
sugars, 18–20
supplements, 105–107
   antioxidant, 63
   banaba leaf, 52
   calcium, 65–67
   chromium, 51
   to control cortisol, 34–36, 37
   dosages, 107
   to enhance thermogenesis, 71
   green tea, 67–69
   herbal, 36
   for metabolic support, 80, 89–91
   synephrine, 69–70
   for thyroid support, 76–77
   vanadium, 51–52
   weight-loss, 63–65
syndrome X, 43–44, 110
synephrine, 69–70

T

theanine, 34, 35, 68
thermogenesis, 9–10, 24, 56–73
   and aging, 57–59
   and calcium, 66–67
   and calorie restriction, 61
   and dehydration, 62
   dietary supplements for, 65–71
   enhancing, 59–63
   and free-radical production, 62–63
   and green tea, 67–69
   and synephrine, 69–70
   and weight-loss supplements, 63–65
thiols, 63
3-S approach, 3
thyroid, 10, 24, 75–77
thyroid-stimulating hormone (TSH), 76
timing of meals, 21–23
trans-fats (trans-fatty acids), 20–21

V

vanadium, 51–52
vegetable oils, 20–21

W

water, importance of, 62, 94
weight-loss plateau, 9
weight-loss programs, 6–7
weight-loss supplements, 63–65, 72, 104
Weight Watchers diet, 41
Weil, Andrew, 21
Willett, Walter, 21

Y

yohimbine, 64–65

Z

Zone Diet, 8, 41

More Hunter House Books

THE ANTI-INFLAMMATION DIET AND RECIPE BOOK: Protect Yourself and Your Family from Heart Disease, Arthritis, Diabetes, Allergies — and More by Jessica K. Black, ND

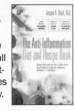

Jessica Black wrote this book for patients who were trying to follow a naturopathic, anti-inflammatory diet. She prepared and tested all the recipes herself, using organic and nutrient-rich foods, eliminating common allergenic foods, and reducing the intake of pesticides and hormones — all of which help to strengthen and heal the body.

The first part of the book explains how the anti-inflammation diet works. The second part contains 125 simple and tasty recipes, from breakfasts, appetizers and herbal teas to soups, entrées, salads, and delicious desserts. Most of the recipes take little time to fix, and include substitution suggestions and health tips. Sample eating plans are included for the summer and winter months, so you can get the added benefit of eating what's in season.

256 pages ... Paperback $16.95 ... Spiralbound $19.95

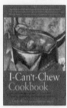

I-CAN'T-CHEW COOKBOOK: Delicious Soft-Diet Recipes for People with Chewing, Swallowing and Dry-Mouth Disorders by J. Randy Wilson

Over 40 million people in the U.S. have chewing and swallowing disorders caused by surgery, cancer, TMJ and dental problems, stroke, Alzheimer's, AIDS, or lupus. Instead of existing on milkshakes, Jell-O, mashed potatoes, and baby food, with the recipes in this book they can get the nutrition their body needs to recover from surgery and disease.

Inside are over 150 recipes for tasty casseroles, soups, and main dishes featuring crab, salmon, ham, and chicken. There are Mexican-flavored entrées, vegetables that are chopped not puréed, and great desserts — food the whole family can enjoy. Each recipe comes with a nutritional analysis, so that you can be sure your meals are healthy and suited to your needs.

224 pages ... Paperback $17.95 ... Spiralbound $22.95

THE *NATURAL* ESTROGEN DIET & RECIPE BOOK
by Lana Liew, MD, and Linda Ojeda, PhD

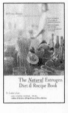

This book is for women who want natural alternatives to hormone replacement therapy (HRT). **Part One** discusses research findings on women's menopausal health and how plant estrogens can alleviate symptoms of menopause. **Part Two** provides over 100 recipes the whole family can enjoy. Chapters include

* Integrating Natural Estrogens into Your Life
* Appetizers, Snacks, and Pick-Me-Ups
* Salads, Side Dishes, and Main Courses
* Pancakes, Breads, Muffins, and Desserts

Includes a glossary and resource section, and nutritional analysis of all recipes.

256 pages ... Paperback $14.95 ... 2nd Edition

More Hunter House Books

THE NO-BEACH, NO-ZONE, NO-NONSENSE WEIGHT-LOSS PLAN:
A Pocket Guide to What Works *by Jim Johnson, PT*

Starting from a "what works" analysis of studies on weight loss, the author gives you proven weight-loss strategies that can be done at home. He explains

* how to determine your body mass index (BMI) and calorie needs
* whether your weight is threatening your health and why your weight problem may not be all your fault
* how to calculate the percentage of fats, carbohydrates, and protein in your diet

Here is a research-based plan for everyone: failed dieters, parents who want to help overweight children, and all concerned health-care professionals.

144 pages ... 6 illus. ... 7 tables ... Paperback $8.95

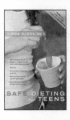

SAFE DIETING FOR TEENS *by Linda Ojeda, PhD*

Living in an image-conscious society where their diets force them to confront with weight issues every day, many teens resort to skipping meals, taking laxatives, or throwing up after eating. But there is a safer and more effective way to get fit and trim. In this handy book Linda Ojeda, a certified nutritionist, offers teens the knowledge they need to create their own diet program. No food is off limits, and teens can adapt the information to their own choices and goals. This book explains

* the math of losing weight, the benefits of exercise
* girls' special diet dilemma and healthy alternatives for snacks and drinks
* the dangers of bad dieting, how to spot a dangerous diet program, and the pros and cons of popular diets such as low-carb and Jenny Craig.

168 pages ... Paperback $14.95 ... 2nd Edition

AWESOME FOODS FOR ACTIVE KIDS: The ABCs of Eating for Energy and Health *by Anita Bean, BSc*

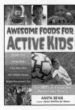

This practical guide contains all the information and suggestions you need to feed growing kids, from kindergarten through high school. Anita Bean explains how to incorporate the best nutrients into your child's diet, how much of each nutrient your child needs, and where they can get it from. Special chapters address the needs of athletes, fussy eaters, overweight children, and eating at school. Includes answers to questions like:

* How do I feed my vegetarian child?
* How much fat should my child have?
* How can I keep my athlete hydrated?
* What should they eat after exercise?

... and much, much more.

224 pages ... 29 b/w photos ... 49 illus. ... 32 tables ... 87 recipes ... Paperback $16.95

To order go to www.hunterhouse.com or call 1-800-266-5592.
Free Media Mail shipping for all personal website orders

More Hunter House Books

THE IBS HEALING PLAN: Natural Ways to Beat Your Symptoms
by Theresa Cheung

Irritable bowel syndrome (IBS) affects 15–20 percent of adults in the U.S. yet, all too often, people affected by IBS choose to suffer in silence. Theresa Cheung's book, packed full of information and help for those suffering from the abdominal pain, bloating, and irregular bowel habits that are the symptoms of IBS, clearly explains the causes and symptoms.

   The healing plan focuses on five key areas: diet, supplements, complementary therapies, stress management, and working with your doctor. Natural remedies include yoga, acupuncture, supplements, stress management, and dietary changes. There is also detailed information about over-the-counter and prescription drugs, their benefits, and their drawbacks.

168 pages ... 9 illus. ... Paperback $14.95

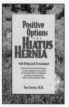

POSITIVE OPTIONS FOR HIATUS HERNIA: Self-Help and Treatment *by Tom Smith, MD*

A hiatus hernia is a common and potentially serious condition that occurs when the upper part of the stomach pushes through the diaphragm, causing a gastric reflux condition (GERD) that is the source of chronic pain for 30 percent of American adults. This book describes how a hiatus hernia comes about, why it could be dangerous, and how to protect yourself from serious developments including esophageal cancer. It describes:

* tests and medical treatments, including drug and surgery options
* self-help, including diet, eating habits, fitness, and stress management

   The clear information will help you to get the treatments and make lifestyle changes you need to manage this poorly recognized but widespread condition and live free of symptoms.

128 pages ... 4 illus. ... Paperback $12.95

POSITIVE OPTIONS FOR LIVING WITH YOUR OSTOMY:
Self-Help and Treatment *by Dr. Craig A. White*

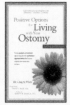

An ostomy is a surgically created opening used to expel waste when the body's normal systems are damaged. This book provides the information you need to deal with the practical and emotional aspects of life after ostomy surgery. Dr. White describes what happens before and during the surgery; how to adapt to wearing an ostomy-care appliance, and how to care for and change it.

   Aware of the long-term concerns of patients and their families, Dr. White provides extensive information on recognizing common emotional reactions, including anxiety and depression, adapting proactively, and knowing when to seek help. Helpful lists and forms provide guidelines for dealing with changes in social interactions, intimate relationships, and sexual activity.

144 pages ... 4 illus. ... Paperback $12.95

To order go to www.hunterhouse.com or call 1-800-266-5592.
Free Media Mail shipping for all personal website orders